Taking the Lead

Kyle P. Meyer · Rob Kramer

Taking the Lead

A Guide for Emerging Leaders
in Academic Medical Centers

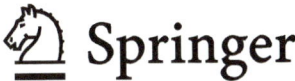
Springer

Kyle P. Meyer
College of Allied Health Professions
University of Nebraska Medical Center
Omaha, NE, USA

Rob Kramer
Kramer Leadership, LLC
Chapel Hill, NC, USA

ISBN 978-3-031-16713-3   ISBN 978-3-031-16711-9   (eBook)
https://doi.org/10.1007/978-3-031-16711-9

This Springer imprint is published by the registered company Springer Nature Switzerland AG
The registered company address is: Gewerbestrasse 11, 6330 Cham, Switzerland

Foreword

You have strong leadership ambitions with a desire to be an extraordinary leader who can influence others to make needed transformational change in health care. Throughout the disruption resulting from the recent pandemic and social unrest, your organization has largely been successful in fulfilling their strategic vision. However, you recognize the imminent transition of your predecessor and other staff changes due to the "great resignations" will leave a knowledge gap that will be an added challenge as you prepare to take on your new leadership role. These concerns, expressed by many related to leadership "knowhow" and courage, generate deep conversations when I wear my executive coaching hat as Division Chair of HR Leadership and Talent Development at Mayo Clinic.

Throughout my experience in human resources development at academic medical centers, I have observed emerging physician (and other health care) leaders, some eager and others reluctant, with some not well equipped for leadership responsibility as an early careerist. The lack of readiness is usually related to limited leadership experience, exposure, or education. Until recently, as would be expected, health professionals' education has been focused primarily on medical and health-related curricula versus leadership development. Without requisite leadership knowledge, skills and ability, health professionals moving into leadership roles may not know what to do as a new leader and, as a result, may struggle in developing strategies and building teams while executing plans and maintaining relationships.

In discussions with coaches and talent development practitioners supporting leaders across various industries in private and public sectors, as well as not-for-profit and for-profit organizations, a commonly shared human resource strategic focus area is developing leaders for the future. There is hyper focus on accelerating the development process. For emerging physicians and other health profession leaders, this acceleration involves unique challenges as they balance patient and leadership needs. Patient needs are aligned with the emerging leader's passion and purpose, and the leadership needs are aligned with the leader's aspiration to have a meaningful impact on the system that supports the patient. The new leader's inherent value of altruism lessens the tension between these two critical needs and motivates the emerging leader to learn the art of leadership.

Even with this altruistic objective, leadership is not easy—it is hard. There will be moments of doubts and times of crisis. For these reasons, leadership requires a strong commitment and purposeful development. Leadership development includes clarity of the leadership role and responsibility, awareness of personal strengths and opportunities related to competencies associated with the role, and measurable goals. The process of becoming an extraordinary leader takes time and intentionality. To move to the next level, dedicated time will be required to attend learning programs, invest in coaching, network internally and externally, assess environments, and read articles and books.

Taking the Lead: A Guide for Emerging Leaders in Academic Medical Centers is "just what the doctor ordered" for both emerging and existing leaders—physicians, health professionals, scientists, administrative leaders—who want to increase their effectiveness. This incredible book addresses the core capabilities that will help ensure a successful leadership journey in academic medical centers. It is a practical and actionable guide to gain leadership insight and perspectives in the context of your organization, your team, and yourself as a leader. Meyer and Kramer understand "leadership can be all time consuming" and, as trusted guides, they share invaluable wisdom in a conversational tone that is easily digestible, with an excellent list of do's and don't's, coaching questions, and resources within each chapter. Keep this book as a ready reference to maximize your potential and add ongoing value to your organization, the patients you serve, and the people you lead.

Turn the page and take the lead.

Division Chair, Human Resources, Assistant   Priscilla Gill, EdD, MBA, PCC
Professor of Health Care Administration
Mayo Clinic College of Medicine
and Science
Rochester, MN, USA

Preface

We, the authors of this book, propose that "leadership" has been with us literally from the dawn of time. In fact, we believe leadership is an inherent characteristic of the human experience. The initial conversation between the first two speaking human beings, we imagine, went something like this…

Human #1: *"OK, so now whatta' we do?"*

Human #2: *"Follow me."*

And thus, leadership was born!

All kidding aside, the purpose of this book is to provide skill development guidance for anyone interested in or recently appointed to a leadership role in an academic medical center (more on this in Chap. 1). We say "skill development" as we believe leadership can be learned. That is, knowledge and insights can be gained, competencies practiced, and abilities refined, based on learning, experience, and reflection.

However, we also believe that leadership is as much art as science. Which is why it is equally magnificent and vexing. Every leader may acquire the knowledge and competencies to lead, but *how* they apply and refine these tools is the art which often determines the leader's success.

Collectively, we have been involved in a variety of leadership roles for more than 60 years, and have coached, mentored, and developed future leaders for nearly as long. In these roles we have learned, experimented, reflected, failed often, and come back for more. Co-author Kyle P. Meyer traces the beginning of his formal leadership journey to 1977 when he was elected as the president of his physical therapy class. He went on to serve in formal roles as Chief Pediatric Physical Therapist, Director of Clinical Education, President of the Faculty Senate, chair of a national professional committee, president of a regional professional committee, Associate Dean, Senior Associate Dean, and Founding Dean. Along the way, he also served in volunteer leadership positions as President of the PTA, chair of a not-for-profit board, and president of an alumni association.

Co-author Rob Kramer has served in leadership roles in higher education as Senior Leadership Advisor, Founding Center Director, and Department Director; in non-profits as Executive Director; and as a professional Executive Coach, working with clients including hospital CEOs and C-suite executives, academic medical center deans, chairs, and administrative leaders, university presidents, provosts, deans, and other senior academic leaders. He is also the founder and CEO of a successful coaching and consulting firm, leading a team of more than 30 coaches who provide executive coaching and leadership development for senior leaders in higher education, academic medicine, non-profits, and the public sector.

This brief overview of our leadership journeys is not intended for self-aggrandizement, rather, simply to establish some credibility. We want you to know that with each of our respective roles we've acquired invaluable lessons in leadership. These came from knowledge gained through formal instruction, informal mentoring, considerable reading, from coaching and being coached, and by applying knowledge from other fields to the art of leadership.

And we have benefited from wonderful colleagues and mentors who often saw more in us than we saw in ourselves. The list of people we could acknowledge for their contributions to our personal, professional, and leadership development is astonishingly long. These individuals taught, challenged, and more than once, bailed us out!

Our primary goal with this book is to serve you in a similar role. To share our lived experiences as mentors, formal and informal coaches and leaders, teachers, supporters, and guides. It is our sincere hope that our reflections, insights, tools, and ideas will serve as both conceptual and practical guidance for you along your leadership journey.

This book is *not* intended to be a "how to" nor a comprehensive "tour de force" on leadership (although it certainly contains plenty of useful and applicable information). In perusing the table of contents, you likely note that there are no chapters on preparing a budget, strategic planning, or managing personnel issues. Rather, this book represents our collective insights—a book of leadership wisdom if you will. The chapters present a series of leadership themes, derived from our own unique observations and perspectives, our own personal mistakes and growing pains, and our observations of other leaders (both successful and unsuccessful). We have selected themes we find important, both about leadership in general and leading in an academic medical center.

We use the word "theme" deliberately because the content of any given chapter is not wholly about a specific topic, but rather an assembling together of observations, reflections, insights, and tools related to that topic. Our purpose is to provide you with ideas, concepts, and insights that have helped us, and in so doing, our hope is that our experience can inform yours, assisting you in acquiring new skills and different perspectives, avoiding some of the mistakes we made, and becoming the best leader you can be.

A note about our writing style. You'll quickly learn that we're very serious about developing new leaders in academic medical centers, but we're also pretty informal. We believe we can better convey our thoughts in a more conversational style. And we think humor is an important aspect of leadership, and life, so you'll note some subtle (or not so subtle) reflections that are on the "lighter side" throughout the book.

We want to draw your attention to a unique feature of the book. We've ended each chapter with a section entitled, "How do I get started?" It includes a "virtual" executive coaching session consisting of relevant questions, not unlike the guidance you might receive from an executive coach. The questions are designed and arranged to facilitate your continual reflection on, and application of, the key concepts within the chapter. We encourage you to return to them often, as you will generate different answers and new insights as you continue to gain leadership experience. We also conclude each chapter with additional resources, entitled "Curious to learn more?" to assist you in building your leadership understanding and knowledge.

Thank you for your passion to lead and for letting us be a part of your journey!

Omaha, NE, USA   Kyle P. Meyer
Chapel Hill, NC, USA   Rob Kramer

Acknowledgments

We would like to thank Phillip M. Pierorazio, MD, Chief, Section of Urology, Penn Presbyterian Medical Center for engaging us in a formative conversation that shaped the content of Chap. 4. We would also like to thank Jesse A. Meyer, PhD, Chief Development Officer, Saint Ignatius College Prep, and Brian Anderson, MEd, MBA, Senior Director of Development, University of Nebraska Medical Center, University of Nebraska Foundation for their guidance and feedback on the development of Chap. 14.

Special thanks to Richard Lansing, Editorial Director, and the team at Springer for their incredible support and skills in making this project a reality.

Contents

About the Authors

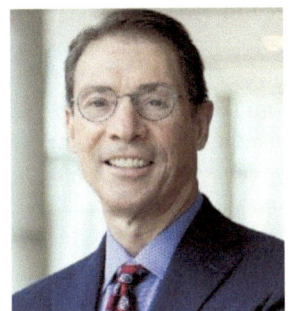

Kyle P. Meyer, PhD, MS, PT, FASAHP Upon earning his Bachelor of Science degree in Physical Therapy from the University of Nebraska Medical Center (UNMC), Dr. Meyer began his career—that now spans over four decades—as a physical therapist. He practiced pediatric physical therapy for over 20 years and was instrumental in developing the first pediatric physical therapy department at Children's Hospital and Medical Center in Omaha, NE. He returned to his alma mater in 1991 as a faculty member and Director of Clinical Education in the physical therapy program. He has gone on to hold several leadership positions throughout his over 30-year career at UNMC, including Associate Dean and Senior Associate Dean for Allied Health in the College of Medicine prior to being named the Founding Dean of the UNMC College of Allied Health Professions in 2015. Dr. Meyer also holds a Master of Science degree (anatomy) from UNMC, and both a Master of Public Administration and a PhD in Public Administration from the University of Nebraska Omaha. Dr. Meyer was a Credentialed Clinical Trainer for the American Physical Therapy Association (APTA) Clinical Instructor Education and Credentialing Program (CIECP) and the Advanced Credentialed Clinical Instructor Program for 12 years. He served as a member and chair of the national APTA Clinical Instructor Education Board and co-authored the Advanced Credential Clinical Instructor Program. In 2016, Dr. Meyer was elected as a Fellow in the Association of Schools Advancing Health Professions (ASAHP) for his record of demonstrated leadership and significant contributions in allied health. He currently presides as President of the Midwest Deans Association of the ASAHP. College of Allied Health Professions, University of Nebraska Medical Center, Omaha, NE, USA

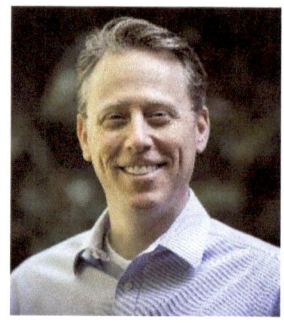

Rob Kramer, MFA, PCC Since 1998, Rob Kramer has provided executive coaching, consulting, and training, specializing in higher education and healthcare leadership and team development. He has served in leadership roles for more than 20 years in academia, including as the founding director of the Center for Leadership and Organizational Excellence at NC A&T State University and as the director of Training and Organizational Development at the University of North Carolina. Rob continues working in faculty leadership development at UNC-Chapel Hill's Institute for the Arts and Humanities. As CEO of Kramer Leadership, he oversees a team of 35 professional coaches across the country, providing executive coaching and leadership development for academic medical centers and higher education institutions. Rob is the author of *Stealth Coaching,* and *Management and Leadership Skills for Medical Faculty and Healthcare Executives* (Springer. 2nd edition, 2020); the latter has been recognized by the United Nations for helping achieve their Sustainable Development Goals for Health and Well-being. He has provided a leadership column for *Advance* healthcare magazine and is a regular contributor of leadership articles for *The Chronicle of Higher Education*. Additionally, Rob has guest lectured at Yale University, the University of Virginia, Duke University, and the University of Colorado, among other academic institutions. Rob did undergraduate studies at the University of Delaware and his graduate studies at the University of North Carolina and UNC-Charlotte. Rob is a Fellow at the Institute of Coaching—McLean Hospital, Harvard Medical School affiliate. He is a Professional Certified Coach (PCC) from the International Coach Federation (ICF), a Center for Creative Leadership coach, and an active member of ICF, the Association of Leadership Educators, and the Organizational Development Network. Kramer Leadership, LLC, Chapel Hill, NC, USA

Part I

Leadership in the Academic Medical Center: Insights and Perspectives

Introduction: Why You Should Read this Book

1

The title of this book is both purposeful and honest. We have worked for most of our professional lives in and with academic medical centers. It is the "site" of much of our collective leadership experience and development. As large, often bureaucratic, multi-mission organizations with competing priorities, academic medical centers represent not only an important form of organization, but a unique form as well (more on this in Chap. 2).

The Need to Develop Leaders

According to the American Association of Medical Schools (AAMC), there are approximately 154 accredited medical schools and more than 400 major teaching hospitals and health systems in the US [1]. These institutions deliver high quality, complex clinical care, serve as the foundation for continuous discovery pertaining to biomedical and clinical research, and educate the next generation of health care providers, not just in medicine, but allied health, dentistry, nursing, pharmacy, and public health.

For their survival and success, academic medical centers need to educate not only the next generation of health care providers, but the next generation of leaders to guide these unique, complex, and in many ways "peculiar" organizations. For academic medical centers to fulfill their highest value to society, they will need outstanding leadership.

The "Emerging" Leader

Our commitment to develop the next generation of academic medical center leaders led us to write this book, specifically for "emerging leaders." There are several general characteristics that define an emerging leader. Such an individual has expressed

K. P. Meyer, R. Kramer, *Taking the Lead*,
https://doi.org/10.1007/978-3-031-16711-9_1

interest in learning about or developing the knowledge and skills to pursue a formal leadership role or trajectory. They are generally recognized by others, peers and superiors alike, as having "leadership potential." Lastly, they are a high performer in one or more missions of the academic medical center (teaching, research, clinical care). As a result, emerging leaders usually have a sponsor or advocate within the organization that provides them opportunities to participate in leadership activities, to begin developing and honing their skills. More specifically, emerging leaders are individuals in the academic medical center who are either preparing to assume a formal "entry-level" leadership role, or who are in their first few years of having assumed such a role.[1] Examples of these roles include Faculty Senate President, Department or Program Director, Division Chief, Department Chair, or Assistant Dean.

One other common characteristic we have observed about emerging leaders is that at least at the outset of their leadership journey, they often do not possess a formal educational background in leadership or administration. As such, as it pertains to leadership, the emerging leader is often left to "figure it out" on their own. As their journey evolves, the emerging leader may choose to pursue formal education and administrative credentials, (e.g., MBA, MPA, MHA), but early "education" on leadership typically involves some combination of "trial and error," faculty development programming, profession-sponsored leadership development training, coaching, and mentoring.

This book is not intended as a substitute for formal academic education in leadership and administration. Rather:

> The goals of this book are to be a resource for the individual in an academic medical center who wants to pursue a leadership role or is within the first few years of assuming that role, and to provide the new leader guidance to enhance their early leadership career, thus establishing a foundation for a successful leadership journey.

As you start exploring the field of leadership, be warned, there is no end of books, lay articles, and academic publications. A Google search on "leadership" offers over five billion entries! And renowned leadership professor Ralph Stogdill famously pointed out back in 1974 that there are almost as many definitions of leadership as there are people who have tried to define it [2]. This pattern has not slowed since, but rather has grown exponentially as colleges and universities around the world continue to expand their leadership faculty, research, and offerings. Since you are at

---

[1] To encompass both conditions of preparing for, or having recently assumed a leadership position, we use the terms "emerging" and "new" to be synonymous throughout the book.

an *academic* medical center, we recommend you begin your journey with a general *academic* understanding of leadership. Review articles on leadership theory and leadership style are a good place to begin (see "How do I get started" at the end of the chapter).

Reading a couple of review articles is not a substitute for a thorough knowledge, but gaining a basic understanding of terms, theories and styles should assist you in establishing a base to begin considering your leadership style and its possible impacts.

What to Expect

We categorized the content of the book loosely into parts, each containing several related chapters. Chapters are structured to provide insights to the topic being discussed, and as we noted previously, end with the section, "How do I get started?" which provides reflection questions and suggested action steps. This structure is designed to be much like working with both a mentor and an executive coach.

Part I examines some of the characteristics of the academic health center (Chap. 2) and presents practical and conceptual considerations for transitioning to a leadership role in this unique environment (Chapters 3 and 4). Additionally, we present a high-level overview of the fundamental work of leaders (Chap. 5), and how the leader can identify and capitalize on their strengths and motivations (Chap. 6).

The goal of these chapters is to establish context, a "starting point" if you will, about the environment in which you will work, the work you will do, and the skills and attributes you bring to the role of leadership. We wanted to provide you some clarity about leadership as a calling in the academic medical center, not simply a job you do. In essence, to help you consider exactly what "you signed up for."

Leaders make decisions every day, all day. It might be said that decision-making is one of the key functions of a leader, and that effective decision-making will determine the success of the leader (and the organization they lead). If you observe leaders for a period of time, you can often discern their decision-making "pattern." A leader's "pattern" brings consistency to the organization and others learn over time what to expect from the leader, even anticipating the decision or adopting a similar decision-making approach (as in, "I wonder what my supervisor would do in this situation?").

Given the importance of decision-making, Part II offers insights into a framework for decision-making (Chap. 7), a caution about decision-making that is somewhat unique to leaders in academic medical centers (Chap. 8), observations and encouragement about the *process* of decision-making (Chap. 9), and decision-making as it pertains to career development and choosing opportunities for growth (Chap. 10).

When people speak of "leaders" they often equate the term to "the boss." Obviously, there are individuals who hold *the* leadership position at *the* top of the organizational chart, the CEO, the President, the Chancellor. But most leaders in big organizations, certainly in academic medical centers, lead a subunit of the organization (e.g., college, department, program, etc.). This is true for the emerging leader, as well. As such, emerging leaders have at least one supervisor, if not multiple.

Part III explores three themes we believe are too often overlooked in the preparation of leaders in academic medical centers, but critical to their success. These topics include interacting effectively with your supervisor (Chap. 11), understanding (and following) the chain of command (Chap. 12), and the value of working "behind the scenes" (Chap. 13). In addition, we examine two specific and important activities for leaders in academic medical centers, philanthropy (Chap. 14) and accreditation (Chap. 15). The goal of these chapters is to give you some insights on how you can improve the effectiveness of your leadership *within* the network that is the large academic medical center.

After the day-to-day importance of making effective decisions, serving as "change agent" is arguably one of the most important roles of the leader. We take this up in Part IV (Chap. 16), along with other leadership challenges, including negotiation, mediation, and conflict resolution (Chap. 17), and crisis management (Chap. 18). This section closes with a topic that we have seen written very little about in leadership, but one that presents a unique challenge to the leader, betrayal (Chap. 19).

The epilogue (Part V) presents some closing reflections on the parallels between our shared hobby of bicycling and leadership (Chap. 20), pointing to the value of having other interests, and taking care of yourself as a leader.

How Do I Get Started?

This book provides an initial footing into the realm of academic medical center leadership. It is organized to make finding the topics you need easy, much like a resource guide. Consider it your initial field book or roadmap. As you begin your leadership journey, we encourage you to talk to trusted colleagues who have also moved into leadership, to learn from their experiences. You may also find it helpful to identify a mentor(s) to help you with specific aspects of your leadership skill development. Above all else, have patience. You will make mistakes as a leader. Forgive yourself, learn from the experience, and try again.

Coaching questions to ask yourself:
- Why am I interested in leadership?
- What do I hope to accomplish as a leader?
- What concerns me most about taking on leadership roles/responsibilities?
- Whose help/support (both professionally and personally) do I need as I begin my leadership journey?

Curious to learn more?
1. Khan Z, Nawaz A, Khan I. 2016. *Journal of Resources Development and Management*, Leadership Theories and Styles: A Literature Review. 16(1), pp. 1–7. Available at https://www.iiste.org/
2. Van Wart M. 2013. Lessons from Leadership Theory and the Contemporary Challenges of Leaders. *Public Administration Review*. Available at https://doi.org/10.1111/puar.12069

References

1. Fisher K. Academic Health Centers Save Millions of Lives. Medical centers save lives. 2019. https://www.aamc.org/news-insights/academic-health-centers-save-millions-lives#:~:text=But%20there%20is%20one%20important,teaching%20hospitals%20and%20health%20systems.
2. Stogdill RM. Handbook of leadership: a survey of theory and research. New York: Free Press; 1974.

The Milieu of the Academic Medical Center

2

As a starting point, we think it's important to examine some key characteristics of the academic medical center as an organizational structure, and to consider the influence the unique features of this structure may exert on *how* and *how well* a new leader applies their craft.

Some General Observations about Academic Medical Centers

An interesting feature of an academic medical center is that it is not one thing. Rather, a given academic medical center (as an umbrella term) is made up of tens, if not hundreds of units necessary to fulfill the teaching, research, clinical care, and community engagement missions of the institution. The differences between units are not simply based on functional purpose and role in achieving the mission(s). Each unit has a different leader, members, history, culture, and perspective about its role and value to the organization. To add to the complexity, these elements are not static; they change over time as the leaders and members change and as the work of the unit evolves.

Another interesting factor about the academic medical center's unique organizational structure is the presence of several paradoxes. Academic medical centers are amazing places to work, filled with a certain "buzz." The work is exciting, inspiring, and even legacy building. But sometimes, despite their focus on discovery, their emphasis on team-based care, their foundation in altruism, and their purpose to advance health and wellness, they can be:

- slow to embrace change
- incredibly competitive
- extremely political
- less mindful of the impact of workload and stress on their employees

K. P. Meyer, R. Kramer, *Taking the Lead*,
https://doi.org/10.1007/978-3-031-16711-9_2

These organizational characteristics can make leading in the academic medical center simultaneously gratifying and frustrating.

Multiple Missions

Perhaps the most obvious characteristic of the academic medical center is its concurrent focus on the multiple missions of (typically) education, research, healthcare delivery (clinical care), and community engagement. These missions are theoretically "equally weighted," although they may not be equally distributed. Since some missions generate more revenue than others, competition for resources can and does occur within units, and leaders often grapple with how to effectively embrace (fulfill) the multiple missions. To add to the complexity, a given unit may be asked to fulfill a mission at the unit or organizational level without direct funding, resulting in the infamous "unfunded mandate."

Without going into great detail about any given budget model, as an emerging leader you will need to understand how (and if) these various missions are achieved in your unit, which generate revenue, and how that revenue is distributed to support all of the various missions. The clinical mission generally produces the greatest revenue, allowing for a redistribution of funds to support the other missions. The expression, "no margin, no mission" conveys this reality.

Leaders must learn to collaborate with their unit members, as well as with members of other units, to deliver on these missions. Thus, a few core leader responsibilities include, determining the primary mission(s) of a given unit (or their relative order of importance), aligning and balancing the missions in accordance with the budget, making sure the goals of the unit align with the academic medical center's goals and strategy, and learning and leveraging the talents of the unit's faculty and staff.

Shared Governance

Academic medical centers are a different breed of organization to be sure, not just because of the varied missions, but largely because of the *academic* component of the medical center, which is grounded in the concept of *shared governance*, as defined here:

> Shared governance has come to connote two complementary and sometimes overlapping concepts: giving various groups of people a share in key decision-making processes, often through elected representation; and allowing certain groups to exercise primary responsibility for specific areas of decision making [1].

Shared governance is most often considered for its value in participation and/or contributions of ideas or feedback across a range of stakeholders, *prior* to a decision being made. In other words, shared governance tends to focus on the "input" side of the equation (and less on the "output" side). Once input has been obtained, a single individual (usually the senior leader), or in some instances a small group of leaders, are left to make a final decision. Hence, on the path to a verdict, the final decision maker is often left to sort out a wide breadth and depth of stakeholder input, and then put it into action. Ultimately, "true shared governance attempts to balance maximum participation in decision-making with clear accountability." [1].

There are a couple of interesting aspects of shared governance that bear further consideration. First, stakeholders may have different views and perspectives about what the "best" decision should be, and any given stakeholder group is likely to believe their proposed outcome should be the one most highly valued by the leader. Second, while the shared governance model privileges many groups to give input, generally only the leader is accountable for the ultimate decision. And the leader must be prepared that not all stakeholders will be pleased with the final decision. This is a critical distinction: shared governance provides for many participants to give input, but generally those participants do not have formal (final) decision-making authority.

An improper understanding of shared governance, or failure to acknowledge the difficulty in maintaining balance between participation and accountability, can lead people to mistakenly think that the relationship between "the faculty" and "the administration" by the necessity of shared governance, needs or tends to be adversarial. Similarly, those stakeholders who do not obtain their desired outcome may accuse the leader of not listening. This is often a euphemism for "you didn't do what I wanted (or told) you to do." One strategy we have found useful to mitigate this outcome is to be very explicit in providing a preemptive explanation about how you plan to use the feedback regarding any pending, relevant decision.

Develop the habit of carefully ensuring each stakeholder (individual or group) that you appreciate their input and will take it under consideration. Also, *explicitly* tell them that you will be seeking input from a variety of stakeholders and will ultimately need to consider multiple perspectives. Consequently, communicate that while you clearly understand their position, the ultimate decision may not reflect their preference. In the end, it's important to keep the following question close at hand when making decisions as the leader: "Who am I willing to disappoint or upset with my decision?"

"Government Should Be Run Like a Business" ... Or Should It?

There is a condition associated with the academic medical center, especially those that are public, that can have an impact on a new leader's capacity to engage in shared governance. Because public academic medical centers often receive funding from the state budget, a perception can exist (particularly on the part of the lay public) that they are a part of the "government." This view can be associated with the narrative that "government should be run like a business."

We understand that health systems and institutions of higher learning *are* businesses. And we also understand that this perception is too often the result of waste, fraud, or inefficiency; so many of the negative complaints leveled against "government." But to be clear, government is not like private business. In fact, government, including academic medical centers, often do the things that private business cannot (or will not) do [2].

We think it's important to draw the new leaders' attention to this important distinction between the purpose of government and the purpose of private business, because if you try to run your unit solely like a private business you will likely either be frustrated by or violate the very principles of shared governance.

To expand, government is intended to represent and protect a wide range of views and voices and create policy that has the greatest impact for the broadest good. Toward this end, power in government (like in the academic medical center) tends to be distributed, not consolidated. Relatedly, by its very nature, policy development and the accompanying process of gaining stakeholder input takes time, sometimes evoking claims of inefficiency. However, far from the inefficiency associated with incompetence, this "inefficiency" is a purposeful feature of the system, serving to protect against overreach and reducing the likelihood of the rapid advancement of one policy or one group, at the peril of others.

Thus, while we are all for effective, efficient leadership, we encourage the new leader to respect and protect the process. Take the time necessary to work patiently with a broad range of stakeholders and achieve optimal gains for as many as possible. Realize however, that in doing so, you may need to defend your approach against the competing claim that "government should be run like a business."

Incremental Pluralism

The characteristics described above are features of the academic medical center's organizational structure. This structure might be best described as a loosely coupled [3], but highly matrixed organization [4] with parallel, embedded hierarchies.[1] In other words, the academic medical center comprises multiple semi-autonomous entities (e.g., colleges, departments, divisions, etc.), which often work with one another. Resources and authority are generally distributed and decentralized, and each unit has its own unit-based hierarchical structure. However, these units co-exist in the larger system-wide hierarchical structure with specific positions overseeing the entire organization (e.g., Chancellor, Vice-Chancellors, Hospital President and CEO, Vice Presidents, etc.).

Consequently, if you want to succeed as a leader in the milieu of an academic medical center, we recommend you adopt an approach of "*incremental pluralism,*" both as a mindset and as a practical strategy. Doing so will greatly assist you in

---

[1] On a lighter note, the organization is also often referred to as a series of fiefdoms connected solely by a shared complaint about parking.

avoiding a sense of frustration over what can sometimes seem like interminable processes resulting in only marginal gains. More positively, it will help you both appreciate the needs and input of multiple stakeholders, and realize that even small, successive gains over time can result in major changes.

With respect to leadership competencies, incremental pluralism requires skills in advocacy, persuasion, edification, and coalition building, not edicts or closed "board room" decisions. Effective leadership in an academic medical center requires creativity, adaptability, perseverance, and a willingness and capacity to think holistically. It also requires pacing—applying your craft with the long-view in mind. Like the well-known saying, "patience is a virtue," when it comes to being an effective leader in an academic medical center, we might amend this axiom to "patience is the *only* virtue."

From a practical perspective, there are several tactics the leader can employ (patiently) in using incremental pluralism as a strategy. These include:

- Putting forth your objectives and plans well ahead of when you would like the outcome realized—at least a year if introducing a major or voluntary initiative.
- Inviting input and feedback from different stakeholder groups. If the goal is broad, invite diverse input, if the goal is narrower, invite the input from at least two or three expert and/or politically relevant stakeholder groups.
- Working within recognized "proper channels" to introduce your ideas and obtain feedback.
- Using standardized and customary approaches to convey information (e.g., open forums, town halls, Faculty Senate presentations, department meetings, department-wide email updates, etc.).
- Ensuring a feedback loop to let stakeholder groups know what is happening (e.g., who provided feedback, what the feedback indicated, how the feedback was considered and incorporated, or not).
- Bringing back revised iterations of your initiatives to address concerns raised by naysayers and to reinforce backing from supporters.
- Delivering a formal announcement about your decision, especially for major initiatives.
- Planning for a "run up" period, for full adoption and implementation.

Being disciplined to engage these approaches will increase both the likelihood of majority adoption and the quality of the initiative. Failure to use these strategies will likely result in progressive opposition to current, and future, initiatives.

One important key to success in advocacy, persuasion, and coalition building is to create a succinct message with a clear rationale or intended outcome and deliver the same message frequently and consistently (see The Leader's Role as Storyteller section, below). This is often referred to as "staying on message." Being deliberate about this simple tactic can be a big factor in the leader's success.

The Leader's Role as Storyteller

You can't stay on message if you don't have a message. Your message should reflect two or three basic ideas or principles that you intend to convey repeatedly and consistently. For example, your message might be about your vision for the organization, your leadership approach, or the value proposition of your unit. Concurrently, your message might reflect a single concept for the organization to understand about your unit. For example, you want your unit to be known for innovation or collaboration.

Once you've crafted your message, be deliberate about both communicating it often and connecting all communications back to the message. This is a powerful strategy for tying the value of your leadership and your unit to the overall success of the organization. And it will help publicize the success of your unit in a consistent and progressive fashion, both inside and outside the organization.

On the topic of conveying a message, we have observed in our own leadership journeys that within the academic medical center's "idea marketplace," it is not always the best idea that gets advanced. Often it is the best *story* about the idea that ensures its eventual success. For leaders wishing to convey and advance their ideas in the milieu of the academic medical center, particularly in the presence of so many good ideas and competition for limited resources, it can be beneficial to improve their story telling skills.

Generally, the elements of a good story include a premise and setting, a plot, characters, a point of view, and a theme. Keep these in mind as you create your message (story) to ensure you:

1. Connect your idea to your central message (i.e., the theme or narrative arc).
2. Identify the impact your idea will have on specific individuals or groups (i.e., the characters).
3. Select a representative (character) or two from an affected group that you can name and highlight[2].

Lastly, dedicate time and practice to develop and perfect your public speaking and storytelling skills. The key to good storytelling is tying your message to some general *themes*, and even more importantly, being very clear about the probable *impact(s)* of your idea or initiative.

---

[2] Politicians use this strategy regularly, for example when a U.S. President invites a citizen to attend and be singled out at the State of the Union address in order to make a broader point.

How Do I Get Started?
Academic medical centers represent a complex and unique form of organizational structure. Thus, it is critical to understand and implement an approach that supports incremental pluralism. Key components of a leader's success in the academic medical center are to understand the situation and context in which their role is performed, who they need to influence, how to garner support for initiatives, and how to develop and communicate consistent messages.

Coaching questions to ask yourself:
- What challenges me most about working in an academic medical setting?
- Who do I respect in the way they lead within their academic medical center? What are they doing or not doing to be successful? How do they view the context, culture, and politics of the institution? How do they communicate?
- How can I gain insight into the structure and politics in my academic medical center?
- How do I determine what is under my control and what is out of my hands?
- How do I know when to pick battles within the larger institution and when to govern what is in my span of control?
- With whom might I practice my communication and public speaking skills to get useful feedback?

Curious to learn more?
1. Hamstra C & Blakeslee J. Communicating Effectively: Balancing Content and Connection. In: Viera AJ & Kramer R, eds. *Management and Leadership Skills for Medical Faculty and Healthcare Executives: A Practical Handbook*. 2nd edition. New York: Springer Nature: 2020:13–22.
2. Oshry, Barry. 2007. Seeing Systems: Unlocking the Mysteries of Organizational Life. San Francisco: Berrett-Koehler.
3. "'Pearls of Wisdom' for Leadership and Success in Academic Medicine Gathered over a 35-Year Career." The ASCO Post. Accessed August 8, 2021.
4. Schein, Edgar H. 2016. Organizational Culture and Leadership. San Francisco: Jossey-Bass.
5. Simone JV: Simone's Maxims Updated and Expanded: Understanding Today's Academic Medical Centers. North Fort Myers, Florida; Editorial Rx Press; 2012.
6. Smith PO. Leadership in Academic Health Centers: Transactional and Transformational Leadership. J Clin Psychol Med Settings. 2015 Dec;22(4):228–31. doi: 10.1007/s10880-015-9441-8. PMID: 26604205.

References

1. Olson GA, July 23. Exactly what is "Shared Governance"? The Chronicle of Higher Education. 2009. https://www.chronicle.com/article/exactly-what-is-shared-governance/
2. Academic Health Centers: Leading change in the 21st century. Introduction. https://www.ncbi.nlm.nih.gov/books/NBK221676/
3. Weick KE. Educational organizations as loosely coupled systems. Adm Sci Q. 1976;21(1):1–19. https://doi.org/10.2307/2391875.
4. Stuckenbruck LC. The matrix organization. Project Manage Q. 1979;10(3):21–33. https://www.pmi.org/learning/library/matrix-organization-structure-reason-evolution-1837

Transitioning to Leadership in the Academic Medical Center: Conceptual Considerations

3

A typical scenario for the emerging academic medical center leader is one of being hired to guide an existing team or unit. In this situation, the leader brings their knowledge, attributes, vision, and experiences to the role, but will likely "inherit" everything else.[1] Thus begins the new leader's transition journey into their new role.

Although the concept, process, and timespan of the "leadership transition" is somewhat ill-defined, authors often imply that it occurs within the first 3 or 4 months [1, 2]. We agree that there are keys steps the new leader can take in the first few months to effectively establish themselves and get off to a good start (see Chap. 4). We also believe however, that there is a difference between *assuming* the formal role of leader and *transitioning* to leadership, particularly in the complex environment of the academic medical center.

To develop a level of comfort with the transition and begin putting their stamp on the role, the new leader will need to learn about their unit and its members, how to interact effectively with other leaders, and begin understanding the academic medical center system from a new perspective. Relatedly, followers and colleagues will also be learning how to engage the new leader. Given these complexities, we believe the broader process of transition can more realistically take up to a year or more.

Why it Matters to You, the New Leader

During the interview process you likely gained some objective information about the unit you now lead (for example seeing the organizational chart, budget, and latest strategic plan, etc.). You likely also began forming perceptions about the people you met and that you now lead, as well as those you now report to. What is much harder

---

[1] There are occasions when a new unit is created that did not exist before, but this happens with far less frequency. When it does, the leader is likely the first person hired, and the responsibility falls on the new leader to literally create the division or department with the resources provided (or negotiated).

© The Author(s), under exclusive license to Springer Nature Switzerland AG 2022
K. P. Meyer, R. Kramer, *Taking the Lead*,
https://doi.org/10.1007/978-3-031-16711-9_3

to learn during an interview process is the unit's implicit organizational culture and group dynamics. These factors can ultimately be the key to your success or failure as a new leader. Gaining this insight requires an immersive experience, being in the unit for a period of time—a luxury you don't get during the interview process.

But even as new leaders do begin to immerse themselves in their unit, they may encounter another common transition trap. They focus almost solely on what they need to *do*, often missing environmental clues which impact the *doing*. There's a phenomenon in psychology called, "inattentional blindness," [3] that suggests we may miss seeing things that are in plain sight, not because we physically can't see them, but because our attention is directed at something else. The result is that during your leadership transition, you may not fully consider or comprehend your assets, as well as any challenges you face, resulting in unintentional errors that can undermine not only your transition to leadership, but the very success of the leadership role.

There are indicators, however, about what you're walking into, the challenges you may face, and relatedly, your reception as the new leader. Whether you were hired from within the organization or as an outside candidate, key insights can be drawn by taking the pulse of the unit. Examples including learning: how long your predecessor was in the role, how well liked they were, under what circumstances they departed the role, the cultural "health" of the unit, the extent to which your new supervisor knows and is involved with the unit, and to what extent the unit's members view your hiring as a mandate for change. That is the purpose of this chapter, to explore some of these "meta" circumstances under which a leadership transition occurs in an academic medical center. Capitalizing on your knowledge of these conditions will make your leadership experience more gratifying and successful, not just during your transition, but throughout your leadership journey.

Two General Conditions of Hire for a New Leader

There are generally two variables present in any leadership transition, one discrete and one continuous, which can impact both how the new leader assumes their role and their success. What we term the "discrete" variable is the simple condition under which the candidate was selected to be the leader. More specifically, whether the selected leader was an "external" candidate coming from another institution, or an "internal" candidate hired from within the institution.

The "continuous" variable is a little more difficult to define and measure. For our purposes, we call this variable the "state" or "health" of the unit, which may include but is not limited to: (1) the unit's historical success, (2) whether and how much the prior leader was respected, (3) whether the former leader remains in the unit or the institution, (4) the quality of the relationships between the current members of the unit, (5) how the unit is perceived by other leaders and units within the academic medical center, (6) the extent to which the members of the unit are "rowing" in the same direction, and (7) whether the unit has a "prima donna" or a dominant faction.

In considering all of these elements and iterations, the leader will gain an idea about the unit's current "functional" or "dysfunctional" state. If the leader is assuming responsibility for a newly created unit, this information wouldn't be available, but similar information might be gleaned by looking at the organizational health of the broader department or division in which the new unit will be housed.

A new leader's primary challenge is establishing credibility, and relatedly, gaining trust and respect to effectively exercise their new positional authority. This challenge exists whether the leader is an internal or external hire. While challenges exists either way, let's take a more in depth look at relevant factors in both situations.

Assets, Challenges, and Errors Associated with Being an Internal Hire

The primary asset of the leader who is hired from within the organization is that they know the organization well. This may include the organizational culture, the people in the unit, their new supervisor, and the general operations of the unit. The internal hire is likely familiar with the skills, attributes, and tendencies of the members of the unit. Relatedly though, the members of the unit are also familiar with the new leader, which is why this situation can represent both an asset and a challenge.

For the leader hired from within, this challenge might be best summarized by the familiar expression, "no one is a prophet in their own land." While the new leader holds the title of "the boss," members of the unit may continue to engage the new leader in the same manner in which they did in the leader's *former* role. Prior experiences, patterns of interaction, and assumptions about the leader can limit the capacity of the internal candidate to effectively transition from peer to supervisor. The new leader may also feel a sense of loss, as former peers (and oftentimes friends) begin to interact with them differently or less frequently. Former peers may even express that the new leader is no longer "one of us."

Moving from peer to supervisor brings an entirely different set of advantages and complexities. The new leader is about to engage in a process of learning more about their colleagues than they would have ever imagined—the good and the bad. And the team is about to experience their newly promoted colleague in an entirely different way, as their supervisor, but more importantly, their new leader. This transition can be tricky. It would be wise for the new leader to have frank conversations with every member of the unit, inviting an open and honest dialogue about their new role and the potential challenges, and opportunities, of moving from peer to supervisor.

Even with these conversations, initial distancing with former peers is to be expected, and can actually be beneficial and formative. It incentivizes the new leader to turn their attention to building relationships across the institution, expanding their network to include others in similar leadership roles from different units, as well as the members of senior leadership. Individuals at different institutional levels and outside the leader's unit are typically not encumbered by past experiences or perceptions of the new leader, and often prove to be a valuable resource, eager to assist in the new leader's successful transition.

Bear in mind that this initial distancing within the unit typically dissipates, and trust returns, if the new leader performs well. Over time, unit members come to see their former peer as their leader, aided by endorsements and support of others in the institution. All new leaders want to perform well, but the context of peer turned supervisor places added stress on the internal hire. If they meet with early struggles or underperform, unit members will likely feel justified in their non-support, even expressing the view that they were certain all along the new situation wasn't going to work.

The new leader's desire to be viewed by their former peers as the "right choice," might cause reluctance in the new leader to confront former peers who provide early challenges to their new authority. The difficulty can be compounded if the resistor is a senior member of the unit, is a prima donna, is highly regarded, or is considered by others to be an "informal" leader for the unit. New leaders may think things will get better over time as others see them perform well as the leader. What happens more often, however, is that by avoiding these initial confrontations, at best the leader is viewed as endorsing the status quo, or at worst they inadvertently provide more power to the resistor.

By failing to confront or address early challenges, the new leader risks creating a perception they are not courageous and will not be an effective leader. Consequently, early challenges must be dealt with immediately with clear and firm communication or action. This might include difficult conversations with individuals or the entire unit, to clarify roles and expectations regarding performance and behavior. In some instances, it may even require the new leader to institute formal corrective action.

The circumstances of these challenges will dictate the response, but we encourage the new leader not to shirk this responsibility. The manner in which these early challenges are met may very well establish the tenor for the new leader's journey within their unit. One word of caution, however. Leadership reactions or decisions that take the form of sweeping decisions or fiats will likely generate unnecessary resistance, as they will be viewed as arbitrary, done solely for the purpose of demonstrating power and not dealing directly with the problem person(s). The new leader will do well to pick their battles wisely.

Assets, Challenges, and Errors Associated with Being an External Hire

One of the principal assets of a new leader hired from outside the organization is the possibility for the infusion of new ideas. These may generate from the both the new leader's experiences at their former institution, as well their expanded network of regional and national contacts. Anticipation about new ideas and a fresh perspective is often a reason for hiring a leader from outside, as it can often bolster morale and generate renewed enthusiasm and engagement from the unit members.

The new external leader will not typically have to deal with prior work relationships and perceptions by unit members. However, some members may withhold their support until they feel the new leader has proven themselves worthy and valuable. This nuance can be further complicated by disappointment or jealousy from any internal members who may have also applied for the role and not been selected.

While the new external leader may be confronted by the same challenge of establishing leadership authority, they are prone to make a different error in response. They often move too swiftly in demonstrating their authority or expertise. In other words, they may feel pressure to demonstrate their value, putting their leadership stamp on the unit. This behavior manifests in the introduction of rapid and widespread change, often with limited consideration for the current members, the unit's unique history, and its values and existing culture.

As noted above, one of the biggest assets a new external leader has is their past experience at different institutions. The goal is to bring this experience along with best practices to their new institution. However, the new leader should not try to implement them "overnight" nor force their new institution to be like their former one.

Unit members will appreciate the new leader's experience, but they do not want to hear how much better the leader thinks their former place was to their new unit. The comparisons may send a message of disrespect, suggesting things are "wrong" with the unit or proposing the new leader isn't interested in learning about the unit. The new leader's action may be interpreted as them saying, "I've already figured it all out. Build a bridge and get over it, we're moving on." Such an approach not only creates unnecessary distress, but also an ineffective paradox. Mindlessly exerting leadership authority can create unnecessary resistance.

A related error for the externally hired leader, particularly one highly recruited and touted for their previous success, is making the unit changes about themselves. Consider for example a new leader who is hired for their research prowess at a former institution. They enter the new unit and quickly reorganize the entire structure to support their research. This person will probably not be met with great support by members of the unit. In this instance, it would be wise for the new leader to be very clear on their new role: to lead the unit to *collective* new achievements in research, and not to create a situation that singularly supports the advancement of their own career.

To be clear, there is nothing wrong with introducing change, especially that which improves the organization's desired outcomes. The trick for newly hired external leaders is to avoid comparisons and allow sufficient time to get to know the members of the unit and the unit's culture. Only then should the leader begin to introduce more incremental changes, giving members appropriate time to understand the rationale for change and to make necessary adaptations.

Two Transition Challenges for the Internal or External Hire

There are numerous other challenges that the new leader faces as they navigate this important transition phase, whether they are hired from within or without. We have chosen to highlight two, as they occur most predictably in the academic medical center. If successfully managed, however, they can be catalysts for the new leader's success.

The first situation involves the former unit leader stepping down but remaining in the unit, returning to other full-time commitments (i.e., returning to a faculty position). Having a former leader in the department can be a tremendous asset, helping the new leader get established for success. Sometimes, however, the new leader may find themselves being haunted by the "ghost of leader past," especially if the former leader was well respected. Unit members will likely compare the new leader to the former leader and continue looking to the predecessor for guidance.

Self-aware former leaders who remain in the unit generally recognize their impact on the new leader and take steps to mitigate any negative consequences, principal among them publicly and routinely endorsing the new leader. However, if the former leader is not savvy enough to direct their colleagues back to the new leader, they may set up a large schism among the unit's members. The former leader should avoid giving the new leader advice in public, assuming key decision-making roles in the unit, or giving too much direction to unit members. These behaviors can unintentionally undermine the new leader. In the rare situation in which the former leader is purposefully creating factions within the unit, the emerging leader will need to have a difficult conversation with the former leader, and perhaps the entire unit, to communicate expectations clearly and explicitly. In extreme cases, a temporary leave or reassignment to another unit may be required to decrease the former leader's influence.

The second challenge that can impede a successful transition is inheriting a unit with a toxic member or faction, and the accompanying dysfunctional behaviors that result. For a new leader to be maximally effective and fully realize their vision, this situation must be dealt with as soon as possible during the leadership transition. Otherwise, the new leader can hope for no more than to serve as the caretaker of a continually dysfunctional and insular unit.

The difficulty with a toxic dominant person is that they can be very successful in their own right, bringing considerable funding or other forms of national recognition to the unit. The success of any one member of the unit is not the issue. Rather, it is the dysfunction that ensues if the person demands special treatment or exerts undue influence at the expense of other's success, of effective teamwork, and of engagement across the unit. As Bill Bradley correctly noted, "the success of the group assures the success of the individual, but not the other way around." [4] Excessive competition, jealousy, efforts to undermine one another, unwillingness to work with particular members of the unit, and difficulty retaining members are a few common symptoms that can result from this circumstance.

If the issue revolves around a "prima donna" member of the unit, it is very likely that the unit members already know there's a problem and are fatigued and frustrated by this person's long-standing negative impact. In this situation, the new leader may find the unit members support action being taken. Successfully navigating the "prima donna" to change behavior, or moving them out of the department, may garner huge support from unit members.

Addressing issues such as these is not for the faint of heart. To discipline or remove a disruptive, dysfunctional member of a unit requires considerable investigation, documentation, negotiation, and adherence to procedural guidelines. It is a time-consuming process, and it should never be handled solely by the new leader. If you find yourself in this situation, do not let it "derail" your transition. We recommend that you bring the situation to others' attention and get the help of superiors, Human Resources, Legal, and any other relevant people or units. One word of caution, be mindful not to invest all of your time working to solve this one issue. The unit members need to see that you are still addressing the broader mission and providing direction for the entire unit.

Concluding Thoughts

Leadership transitions by their very nature are change events, often accompanied by great expectations. The new leader brings with them a new vision, enthusiasm, and hope for the future. Properly done, the leadership transition can be a transformational event for a unit, often reenergizing unit members, expanding resources for the unit, and elevating the unit in the organization's collective consciousness.

It can also be a challenging time for the new leader. However, with a proper understanding of the tasks, conditions, and time that accompany a leadership transition in the academic medical center, and equipped with strategies to address these challenges, the new leader can successfully begin a long leadership career.

How Do I Get Started?

Transitioning into a new leadership role is one of the more critical experiences one can have in their careers. With every promotion, the visibility, politics, and stakes increase. To navigate your transition successfully, consider talking to others you respect who have gone through it themselves. If possible, ask one of them to serve as your mentor through the transition process. Also consider hiring a leadership coach (here's a tip, request funding for a coach in your start up package). Having this confidential confidant is crucial to safely discussing the challenges and opportunities you face, with someone outside the organization, who can give you an impartial perspective and help champion your success. Consider having the coach conduct a 360 assessment for you after 9–12 months on the job. It is a great way to get confidential, honest feedback on your early performance. Lastly, upon hire do not run off and begin attending leadership programs. Reasons being are (1) you want to be visible and available for your new team and to learn the new job, and (2) you don't want to inadvertently signal that you feel deficient in your leadership abilities. Save leadership development programs for year two on the job.

Coaching questions to ask yourself:
- Who do I know and respect for how they navigated their leadership transition?
- What do I need to learn, understand, and do in my first 90–120 days on the job? Who can help me sort this out?
- What strategies do I need to bring with me into this new role, and what behaviors do I need do leave behind?
- What do I need to do to help *others* be successful in my new unit?
- How can I best learn the culture and the people in my new unit?
- What are my highest aspirations for this new role?
- Who do I need to go to if I struggle or not know how to handle an issue?

Curious to learn more?
1. Bean, K. (2015, August 25). Administrators Are People, Too. Inside Higher Ed; Inside Higher Ed. https://www.insidehighered.com/views/2015/08/25/why-professors-shouldnt-view-administrators-such-disdain-essay
2. "From Physician to Physician Leader: Developing Your Skills for Success." Harvard T.H. Chan School of Public Health, Harvard University, 24 May 2018, https://www.hsph.harvard.edu/ecpe/physician-leader-skills-success/.
3. Watkins, M. (2003). *The first 90 days*. Harvard Business Review Press.
4. In Support of Those Who Take the Leap Lessons on Leadership Transitions from the Open Society Foundations' New Executives Fund. September 2021. Available at https://www.opensocietyfoundations.org/uploads/31d2bc8b-bf92–4457-8c13-f7317a30f85b/in-support-of-those-who-take-the-leap-top-advice-for-the-new-executive-directors-from-their-peers-20211019.pdf

References

1. Watkins MD. The first 90 days: proven strategies for getting up to speed faster and smarter. Harvard Business Review Press; 2013.
2. Bradt G, Check JA, Lawler JA. The new Leader's 100-day action plan: how to take charge, build or merge your team, and get immediate results. Wiley Publishing; 2016.
3. Perera A. May 21, 2021. Inattentional blindness. https://www.simplypsychology.org/inattentional-blindness.html
4. Bradley B. Life on the run. 1976. New York, NY: Random House; 1984.

Transitioning to Leadership in the Academic Medical Center: Practical Considerations

4

The cultural norms of the academic medical center prize expertise. Whether related to health professions, graduate education, or clinical care, the expectation is to have the answers, know what you're doing, exude self-assurance, and not display uncertainty.

Confronted with this standard, a common struggle as you enter leadership is challenges with confidence (and if you are not lacking in confidence, it is likely time for a reality check as you may have blind spots about your leadership acumen). Most often the struggle is internal, as the initial excitement of being hired gives way to you, (1) questioning whether you have what it takes to succeed, or (2) having intermittent performance worries. These may manifest in concerns about how well you're doing, whether you're moving too slow or too fast, and whether you said or didn't say the right thing. Alternatively, sometimes the challenge comes from external sources, as in reticence of new followers to demonstrate confidence in you, or others in the organization "testing" your leadership poise and abilities.

The good news is that if you have experienced these feelings or circumstances, you're already more prepared than you think. It takes three things for someone to successfully move into a formal leadership role: preparation, attitude, and opportunity. You evidently exhibited the first two in your career development to date. The person that hired you likely has seen them, and thus provided you the opportunity to lead. So, while it's normal to experience some personal trepidation when assuming a new leadership role, know that whoever hired you already sees your skills and potential even if you don't, and that it may take some time for you to gain your footing in the role.

Every emerging leader's journey is different, but each has one shared goal: avoid the bad beginning. To get off to a good start in your leadership journey we offer several practical keys for you to consider. A chapter could be dedicated to each of these keys, but here we will present a brief list of "do's and don'ts," providing you some action steps and a solid foundation to support your early leadership success.

© The Author(s), under exclusive license to Springer Nature Switzerland AG 2022
K. P. Meyer, R. Kramer, *Taking the Lead*,
https://doi.org/10.1007/978-3-031-16711-9_4

DO Understand Your New Role

Many individuals who come to leadership in academic medical centers do so having exhibited a high level of competence related to the various institutional missions - clinical care, teaching, research, and service. As a new leader, you might have a tendency to believe you can rely on your current skills and instincts in one or more of these areas to succeed in your new leadership role. For starters, let's address that perception.

As we noted above, as a clinician, teacher, and/or researcher, your role was primarily to be the expert, to have and dispense the answers. As leader, however, your role changes immediately. You now need to listen, coach, support, develop, and advocate on behalf of those you lead. One of the biggest challenges for individuals moving into leadership in the academic medical center is the realization they are going from a career that's been about *their* success, to a career that's about the success of *others*. This doesn't mean you have to totally sacrifice your own career, but you will need to adapt your mindset to the primary purpose of your new role: leading.

Part of this adaptation is to accept that you no longer have every answer. In fact, you probably shouldn't know every answer. If you think you do, it will likely be to your detriment. Rather, your new role is more that of "broker." You need to know, or learn, where to find the answers, as well as how to guide others to find their *own* answers.

Another aspect of understanding your role is to "count the cost" of leadership. Individuals assuming formal leadership roles in academic medical centers have generally worked in the environment for some time. So, they are used to hard work and long hours. But leadership is a different kind of hard work. It is not just time-consuming; it can be all-consuming. While it can be immensely rewarding, even exhilarating, it can also be gut wrenching and lonely. We don't want to be too melodramatic, but when emerging leaders fail, it's often because they didn't fully consider the extent of the commitment required to be an effective leader. Of course, how could they if they'd never been one?

DO Clarify Expectations (for Others and Yourself)

One important way to get your leadership journey off to a good start is by establishing clear expectations. Leaders tend to think of this as defining *their* expectations for the members of their unit, but keep in mind, your followers will also have expectations of *you*, as will your supervisor(s). In addition, as you begin to exert your leadership influence and interact with members of your unit, you will create shared cultural expectations about how the unit will function, what it values, and how its members will behave.

Let's begin with the values and expectations you hold for yourself. Clarifying these to your followers will demonstrate your authenticity and let them know that you will hold yourself accountable to be an effective leader. Let the members of your unit clearly understand what you perceive your role to be, how you delineate your duties, and what you plan to prioritize and measure.

Clarify your leadership philosophy and style, which are different but related concepts. Your leadership *philosophy* is essentially your "world view" about leadership. It is a succinct expression of your perceptions of the purpose of leadership, and the primary role(s) of the leader. Leadership *style* is how you personalize your philosophy, and model it through your daily behaviors.

For example, if your leadership philosophy is that the primary purpose of the leader is to create opportunities for others to succeed, you might do this by meeting routinely with your team to discover their needs and career aspirations. As an expression of your personality, you may have an "open door policy" for these types of discussions. If you're style is more formal, you might set aside time each Friday morning to schedule career advancement discussions. In our opinion, there's no right leadership "style." The key is to be true to your personality and values, and act in ways that are consistent with what you say.

If you have procedural expectations (e.g., "ground rules"), these are good to clarify as well. For example, you will want to be explicit about the purpose, frequency, and structure of meetings; what someone should do if they have a problem; how, when, and why you plan to solicit input or feedback about the unit; and how and when you plan to communicate to the unit.

Establishing expectations ahead of time will provide clarity and a transparent understanding among all the members of the unit. It will also begin the process of trust building and go a long way toward decreasing the unease sometimes associated with "getting a new boss." As members of the unit increase their interactions with you and with one another in accordance with your expectations, a collective unit culture will begin to emerge over time that "institutionalizes" the values and accompanying member behaviors.

We recommend you also invite your direct reports to provide their expectations of you. This tactic sends the message that you are interested in their needs, value their input, and sets an encouraging tone for team engagement. You can then collate the feedback into themes (see Table 4.1) and refer to the list periodically to make sure you continue being mindful of these guiding expectations.

Table 4.1 Example of essential expectations a team provides their new Dean

Representation
- The Dean should be the primary ambassador for the college, serving both to provide information and to advocate on behalf of the college.
- The Dean should be the primary link between the various department chairs, section chiefs, and program directors.

Personnel administration
- The Dean should be a good supervisor for the college's associate and assistant deans and department chairs - providing helpful and regular communication, clear expectations, guidance, feedback, support, and recognition.
- The Dean should make personnel and fiscal decisions that are in the best interest of the college.
- The primary outcome for the Dean is the empowerment of college leadership.

Strategy Development & Implementation
- The Dean should develop a shared vision and strategy for the college's advancement.
- The Dean should maintain current knowledge of trends in health professions education, engage in network-building activities at the national level, and develop a strong administrative infrastructure necessary for the advancement of the college.
- The Dean should promote an atmosphere of collegiality and support and engage in continual environmental assessment and quality improvement.

Resource administration
- The Dean should ensure the operational stability and fiscal solvency of the college and its constituent departments and units.
- The Dean should procure the resources necessary to secure the college's goals and desired outcomes, as well as the resources required to achieve new strategic initiatives for advancing the college.
- The Dean should engage in ongoing development activities for the good of the college.

DO Establish a Cabinet

Your cabinet is your own leadership team with whom you will work most closely. There is no magic time frame for establishing your cabinet, but you'll probably start to appoint this group in the first three to six months of assuming your role. If you are assuming leadership of an existing unit, it's very likely a cabinet already exists. These are generally members of the executive team, consisting of persons responsible for specific functions of the unit (e.g., budget, academic affairs or residency program, clinic operations, human resources, etc.). It is certainly your prerogative to arrange this team to meet your needs and the needs of the unit. You may choose to add a member or two, or you may inherit a situation that requires you to fill a position or two. If a formal team exists, we advise against making any changes for several months until you have gotten to know the players, understand how the team functions, and assess where (if any) there are gaps in performance or need.

One critical member we believe must be on your cabinet is the individual responsible for financial affairs. We find that the number one concern most new leaders have about assuming their role relates to the budget. While leaders with a research background may have experience in creating and managing grant budgets, the comprehensive budget process at most academic medical centers is often more complicated.

Academic medical centers employ a variety of budget approaches or models, from incremental, "historical" approaches to responsibility-based budgeting to zero-based budgeting. Many new leaders are unfamiliar with budget models, strategic budget planning, and budget accountability or reconciliation approaches. In addition to learning from the finance officer/director on your cabinet, it may also be useful to consider taking a budget and finance class through your local business school or through one of many online courses for new leaders.

Please note, the presence of a formal cabinet does not preclude you from creating an informal circle of trusted advisers (sometimes referred to as a "Kitchen Cabinet"). We recommend keeping the group relatively small and including individuals from both within and outside your unit, and maybe even outside your organization. For example, a mentor at your former employer, a "senior" individual at your current institution who has been in your same role for a number of years, or a group of individuals in a similar role to yours for 2 to 3 years or more (at your or other institutions) can provide a nice "mix" of experience and support for a new leader.

Unlike the formal cabinet, members of the Kitchen Cabinet may never even meet together. This small group of advisors is intended for your development, for you to "bounce ideas off," and to give you honest feedback about your ideas and aspirations. Some new leaders find working with an executive coach to also be valuable, in place of, or in addition to a Kitchen Cabinet.

DO Hire a Good Administrator

Most units in the academic medical center have a primary manager or administrator who oversees and directs day-to-day operations. With respect to your eventual success as a leader, an effective administrator can be a "make or break" person. You need to find an administrator who understands your vision, supports your work, protects your time, and generally looks out for your best interests.

The "network" of unit administrators in the academic medical center is often the behind-the-scenes group that can truly get things done, so it is important to also have a unit administrator that is trusted and well respected by others who serve in similar roles in different units. If and when you have the opportunity to hire your administrator, be deliberate, take your time, and choose wisely.

The more typical situation, however, is that you will "inherit" the current unit administrator. If this individual is informative, transparent, and collegial, particularly if they have been in the role for some time, they can be an invaluable asset for a successful transition to your leadership. Spend time getting to know your administrator and be open to listening to their advice.

However, if you find yourself with an administrator who is not open or is still embracing the tenure of the former unit leader, be alert to forms of resistance, especially if you attempt to introduce early changes. Resistance may come in the form of your administrator telling you, "This is the way that has always worked best," or "This is the way we've always done it." These statements could very well be true. They may also indicate a lack of understanding about an actual process, or an unwillingness to change. Stronger resistance may take the form of undermining your leadership, stirring up rumors, and poor or limited work performance.

As you begin your new role you will be well served by establishing and clarifying your relationship with your new or inherited administrator. Building trust and a solid working relationship with this person will be one of the biggest keys to your success.

DO Focus on Developing this Important Skill

In an academic medical center, another key to the success of any leader or unit is often the quality of the relationship with *other* leaders and units. This may be within your academic medical center, with other healthcare institutions, or with community organizations. You may already know or possess some of the tools that will allow you to be successful in engaging others, even if you don't know them as "boundary spanning" skills. Boundary spanning has been defined as the "capability to create direction, alignment and commitment across boundaries, fields, or sectors to achieve a higher vision or goal." [1, 2] This involves "optimizing relationships between a leader's span of control and the departments, organizations, communities, and/or broader networks within which it operates." [3].

One way we recommend you can begin the work of establishing a broader network is to invest in identifying and visiting stakeholders. We recommend you engage in a networking "tour" within the first few months of beginning your tenure as leader. A simple introduction and invitation to consider future partnership opportunities can go a long way in establishing your credibility, identifying you as a "team player," and sending the message that you are open to innovation and new or renewed organizational relationships. It can also give you the opportunity to learn first-hand what other units and organizations think of yours, giving you a sense of which relationships might need repair, and which you can begin to rely on immediately.

Becoming effective at boundary spanning will enrich your ideas, expand your reach, and enhance your likelihood for success. Your ability to engage and influence a broader network of stakeholders will multiply your impact and serve as the key to your ultimate success.

DO Expect and Respond to Early Leadership Challenges

As a leader you should expect challenges. In fact, we argue that you should invite them. We are referring to times when you may be legitimately questioned, challenged about a decision, or asked to provide rationale for a selected course of action. This happens (as it should) with some degree of regularity in the normal course of doing your work as an academic medical center leader.

Sometimes challenges come in other forms, however. We are referring to a challenge that clearly has the goal of undermining your work or ability to lead. Common examples include publicly questioning your knowledge or abilities, casting asper-sions on your motives or character, humiliating you to gain an advantage, or misrep-resenting something you said. Thankfully, these types of challenges generally come from a single individual or at most a small group, trying to make a point or gain some advantage. These challenges can occur any time during your leadership jour-ney, but they tend to arise more frequently at the outset, as you work to establish your credibility and gain collaborators, willing followers, and partners (see Chap. 3).

If you've come to a leadership role from within your organization, those doing the "testing" may very well be your former peers. This behavior can be innocent, as your colleagues adapt to your new role, or it can be deliberate, as in attempting to demonstrate that you were not the best choice to lead.

If you are taking on a leadership role having come from another institution, you represent a bit of an unknown entity. Some of the more vocal members of your unit, or those more resistant to change, may feel the need to use the transition as an opportunity to challenge your authority or establish their influence.

In either situation, you may be tempted (or prefer) to ignore the action of these individuals and the resultant confrontation. Don't. Because leadership is often car-ried out in the public arena, members of the organization, including your own team, will observe these challenges. Consequently, you need to recognize that these types of public challenges demand a public response, as the members of your unit will be watching your reaction and forming perceptions about your future capacity to lead. By the way, doing nothing *is* a response and *is* visible to others.

You do not need to be rude, combative, or aggressive. A level-headed and direct response will show integrity, courage, and a willingness to take on conflict appropri-ately. Conversely, withdrawing at the first sight of confrontation in the name of humility, avoiding early confrontation, or any other rationalization, may hurt your credibility as a leader.

Don't misunderstand, there are certainly times when "discretion is the better part of valor," but your role as leader is to convey a confident and consistent message that you have the organization on the right track. Effective leaders are able to state explicitly that they have the determination to succeed, that they believe their vision can propel the organization to new heights, that they have good ideas, and that their approach is productive and effective. It may not be the only approach, but it is cer-tainly one effective method.

DON'T Be in Too Big of a Hurry

The academic medical center has its own unique annual "life cycle," a series of predictable occurrences that happen at roughly the same time each year. For exam-ple, many academic medical centers begin the fiscal year on July 1, which means the strategic planning and budgeting processes likely begin in early spring. Particularly relevant to public academic medical centers, the state legislative process follows a particular calendar cycle. New medical residents and fellows also begin July 1. There is often a buzz on campus in late summer and early fall as new students enter the various education programs. Convocation and commencement usually occur in May, and sometimes in December, as well. Grant applications also often follow specific timelines and cycles.

As a leader, you need to live through an entire annual "life cycle" of events to start to get the rhythm of your role. You've worked in an academic medical center, but in a different capacity, so you will likely encounter novel situations and responsibilities in your first year as leader. It is common for new leaders to be overwhelmed by the amount of new information they will suddenly be exposed to. As an example of this common phenomenon, there is a major research university with an academic medical center that offers a year-long program for new, first year department chairs. The program is affectionately referred to as "chairapy," as it supports these new leaders through their year one, "deer in the headlights," experience of the job.

The second-year cycle will typically be easier as you become more adept at anticipating what will happen and what is expected of you. By year three, you will start to feel like you are settling into the job. This is not an absolute or mandatory timeline, just a general, somewhat predictable observation. Thus, give yourself time to adapt to your leadership role, and mitigate the risk of burnout by not trying to do too much, too soon.

Another aspect of reframing your time can refer to what we call the "time horizon." If your previous role may have been, for example, teaching, your time horizon might have been a few weeks or a semester. Teachers usually create a syllabus for a course based on a semester plan, and then deliver and adjust the curriculum from week to week. On the other hand, if you were primarily involved with clinical practice prior to your transition to leadership, your time horizon might be a few days to a few weeks, as a clinician's schedule often revolves around patient care responsibilities that need to be conducted in that time frame.

We find that an academic medical center leader's time horizon is more like 2 to 3 years. This is often due to the leader being responsible for surveillance of the environment and anticipating pending threats and opportunities. Considering, planning, and implementing new strategic initiatives takes time, as do the processes for acquiring resources and the recruitment of new personnel. Hence, the leader needs a longer time horizon to accomplish their work.

DON'T Assume Others' Problems

We noted earlier that as you transition to becoming the leader, you also transition from having the answers to knowing where to find the answers. This doesn't happen overnight. Many new leaders may struggle with a self-imposed pressure to be action oriented as a strategy to gain credibility and demonstrate that they were the right choice to be leader. A certain type of employee can capitalize on this orientation (sometimes purposefully, sometimes inadvertently). The employee is the one who comes to you with a "very significant problem" that they claim needs your immediate attention, because "only you" can fix it.

Because you believe that being responsive and action oriented is the leader's role, and because you want to demonstrate your effectiveness as a new leader, you may be tempted to earnestly address this request. Don't. Without immediate action, many problems in this category amazingly go away. Not always, of course, but often. Many times, the real owner of the problem uses the transition to project their long-standing issues onto the new leader.

As you mature as a leader, you will come to realize that these situations are seldom the "emergencies" they are described to be. Actually, it is very likely the problem that needs your *immediate* attention has been going on for years. Don't let the purported urgency keep you from carefully gathering the additional information necessary to fully consider the true merits of the concern. Rather than solving the problem, use the situation to provide guidance to the person who brought the concern, so they can learn to solve their own problems. This is one essential component of being an effective leader who coaches.

By the way, this phenomenon of problem offloading occurs regularly throughout all leaders' journeys. So much so, there is a classic Harvard Business Review article [4] that we highly recommend about how to manage it more effectively.

DON'T Listen to this Advice

During your first year as leader, you'll likely receive from one or more senior, sage leaders what is purported to be the "absolute truth" regarding the very foundation of effective leadership. This well-intending advice usually comes in the form of a statement like, "Remember, it's better to be respected than liked." The statement implies there are only two leadership outcomes, and that as a new leader you need to decide which one you will pursue.

This advice is the modernized version and misinterpretation of something said by Niccol'o Machiavelli in his 1532 book, *The Prince,* [5, 6] in which he detailed his views on how to acquire and maintain political power. What Machiavelli actually said (in part) was, "... it is much safer to be feared than loved, if one of the two must be lacking."

Machiavelli was referencing that the most effective strategy for "rulers" to maintain control and avoid overthrow, is noting that humans (who he referred to as "wretched creatures") are more likely to respond to the fear of punishment than the obligation of love.

To be clear, we have no expertise in Italian Renaissance writing, nor are we at war with anyone, nor are either of us a prince. We just wanted to provide you with some context about this quote (and related advice), because we don't think it has a place in modern leadership. We don't disagree with the general sentiment that you will want to be respected as the leader. But we hope you'll agree with us that you won't gain true respect by using the fear of punishment or retaliation. And you certainly won't be able to build important relationships with the members of your unit if you view them as morally bankrupt, "wretched" individuals. We believe that both obtaining the respect *and* building effective relationships with those you lead are mutually beneficial and attainable outcomes. In fact, we think the true measure of leadership greatness is being both respected *and* liked by those you lead.

DO Take Care of Yourself (DON'T Assume the Academic Medical Center Will)

There is an old expression, "no good deed goes unpunished." This paradox plays out daily in the lives of leaders in academic medical centers. Leaders tend to be competitive, goal-oriented, accomplished individuals. Their major goal is generally to successfully develop and advance their unit. Success generally breeds success. But it can also bring more responsibilities to the leader. The more you succeed, and others see your success, the more you will be asked to do. And success has an inexorable appetite. Thus, you must be cautious not to become captured in a trap of your own making. In other words, one of your primary responsibilities as a leader in the academic medical center, is to ensure your own health and welfare.

We highly recommend as you assume your new role, but also throughout your leadership journey, that you consider the impact your leadership commitment has on the other people in your life, as well as on your other roles and responsibilities outside of the academic medical center. Whether you resonate better with the concept of work-life "balance" or work-life "integration," we think most long-term, successful leaders remain mindful of the value of having other interests (see Chap. 20), as well as the need for intermittent periods of rest and recovery. The bottom line is that *you* are responsible to maintain your health and well-being. If you do, we believe you will more effectively engage your roles both at work and beyond.

Concluding Thoughts

The topics above are not intended to be exhaustive. And although we titled the sections, "do's and don'ts," our goal was more to raise your awareness than it was to suggest a "prescription" for success. We wanted to present common situations that confront new leaders, and practical strategies for managing these circumstances should they occur to you. Consequently, we invite you to ponder the topics and consider your personal application and adaptation in light of your experience and your goals.

How Do I Get Started?

Coaching questions to ask yourself:

- As I enter this new role, what are my gaps as a leader I need to be attentive to?
- Who would be beneficial to have as members of my "Kitchen Cabinet"?
- How might I benefit from the help of a leadership coach during my leadership transition? Who do I know that has worked with a coach before to help me understand the value of it and/or to find a coach for myself?
- How can I find out more about the team, culture, and context I have entered (or am about to enter) into?
- What are the critical items I can be looking out for during my first year on the job?
- How comfortable am I managing conflict? If necessary, what do I need to do to adapt my style and/or get better a managing conflict?
- What assumptions am I making as a new leader and in this new role?

Curious to learn more?

1. Ernst, C., & Chrobot-Mason, D. (2010). Boundary Spanning Leadership: Six Practices For Solving Problems, Driving Innovation, And Transforming Organizations. McGraw-Hill.
2. Kramer, R. (2020). Stealth Coaching: A Roadmap to Develop Independent Thinkers, Proactive Problem Solvers, and Exceptional Leaders. Luminare Press.
3. Kramer, R., & Mucha, P. (2018, July 30). 5 Tips on Surviving Your First Year as a Department Head. Chronicle of Higher Education; Chronicle of Higher Education. https://www.chronicle.com/article/5-tips-on-surviving-your-first-year-as-a-department-head/
4. McGregor, D. (2006). The Human Side of Enterprise. McGraw-Hill Education

References

1. Retrieved   from   https://www.rwjf.org/en/library/articles-and-news/2012/07/supporting-boundary-spanning-leadership.html
2. Yip J, Ernst C, Campbell M. Boundary spanning leadership mission critical perspectives from the executive suite. 2009 White Paper by the Center for Creative Leadership. https://cclinnovation.org/wp-content/uploads/2020/02/boundaryspanningleadership.pdf
3. National   Center   for   Healthcare   Leadership.   NCHL   Health   Leadership   Competency   Model   3.0.   Retrieved   from   https://www.nchl.org/research/#NCHL_Health_Leadership_Competency_Model_30
4. Oncken W, Wass DL. Management time: Who's got the monkey? 1999. https://hbr.org/1999/11/management-time-whos-got-the-monkey.
5. Machiavelli N, 1469–1527. The prince. Harmondsworth, England, New York, NY: Penguin Books; 1981.
6. Harrison RP. What can you learn from Machiavelli? 2011. https://insights.som.yale.edu/insights/what-can-you-learn-machiavelli

Strengths and Motivations of the Leader

5

We alerted you at the book's outset not to expect an in-depth overview of the topic of leadership. We've also noted that emerging leaders may not have a lot of exposure to the basics of leadership. In this chapter we will present some foundational aspects to leading well. We focus in particular on the attributes and practices of good leadership.

Most often, new leaders are hired in an academic medical center based on their knowledge, skills, and abilities, often referred to generally as qualifications or "KSA's". These include such things as degree(s), required licenses or certifications, demonstrated competencies, experience (either years or roles or both), accomplishments, etc. What can be more difficult to determine during the interview process is exactly how the leader's personality will manifest in the leadership role.

Thus, the importance of understanding attributes and practices. Attributes are personal traits[1] and characteristics (good or bad) that a leader brings to the role. While often considered inherent, we believe that attributes can be both acquired and improved upon. Additionally, the new leader can develop "practices," intentional, disciplined, and consistently repeated behaviors which support their overall success. As important elements of leadership, attributes and practices have a significant impact on the leader's ultimate success, as they very much shape how a leader leads, and ultimately how their followers will respond.

In this chapter we devote our attention to seven observations about attributes and practices which we believe will be of benefit as you work to shape your own leadership style.

---

[1] Here we use the term "trait" in a generic sense to define recognizable qualities or characteristics. This is different than "trait theory," a leadership model which purports to predict or explain the success of a leader based on the possession of certain, often "inherited," traits.

K. P. Meyer, R. Kramer, *Taking the Lead*,
https://doi.org/10.1007/978-3-031-16711-9_5

Observation #1: Traits—Duality Versus Continuum

Let's begin with a general discussion of traits. People often think about traits from a perspective of "duality." It may be inadvertent, but you will often hear people say things like, "That person is so organized," as if to imply the only other alternative is to be *dis*-organized. To illustrate this "either/or" perspective we've assigned these two opposite traits to each end of a line (see Fig. 5.1a).

In our observations, however, most traits don't manifest in simple dichotomies. We believe leaders would be better served to consider that traits (theirs and others') are expressed along a continuum, with the boundaries of expression represented by their extreme manifestations. Thus, what in a duality model are simply represented as two expressions of a trait, on a continuum model become a myriad of expressions.

To illustrate this concept, in Fig. 5.1b, we have placed the competency, "Organization," at the midpoint of the line where a balanced expression of a trait would be located (think about the fulcrum of a teeter totter) and identified extreme examples of trait manifestations as the line's two endpoints (these may not be realistic extremes, but hopefully you get the point). It's unlikely that anyone is "perfectly balanced," so we've also added a green line to represent where a person might land if their typical tendency is to be "well organized," with a slight preference for control.

Fig. 5.1 Conceptual depictions of "traits". (**a**) Duality model of traits. (**b**) Continuum model of traits. (**c**) Impact of stress on the manifestation of traits

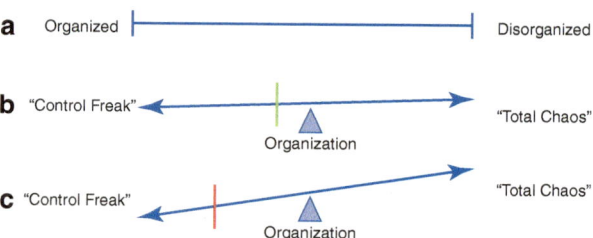

Observation #2: The Impact of Stress on the Manifestation of Traits

When a person is under stress, the concept that traits are manifest on a continuum leads us a second, related, observation. That is, under stress, people tend to move farther *in the direction* of their typical tendency.

To illustrate, if under normal circumstances a person's typical expression of organization tends to favor slightly more control (green line in Fig. 5.1b), under stress they often exhibit behaviors that are *more* controlling (Fig. 5.1c). All this to say, new leaders would do well to examine their own traits and strengths on a continuum. It can help in understanding why they behave the way they do under both typical and stressful circumstances and learn tools to self-correct as needed. Additionally, this self-awareness can assist the new leader in seeing, predicting, and responding appropriately to others when *they* are under stress.

Observation #3: Strengths as Weaknesses

Most of the time we think about strengths as positive traits or characteristics, seeing their value and the good they contribute. Our third consistent observation is that *over*-reliance on a given strength, without an accompanying thoughtful consideration of the unintended consequences, may (paradoxically) diminish the impact of the strength.

For example, according to a popular assessment tool, one of author, Kyle's, strengths is recognizing potential where perhaps others can't. He is both in a constant pursuit of excellence and has the capacity to help others achieve excellence. This sounds like a great skill to have, and who would ever consider it an impediment to effective leadership? Well, what Kyle discovered over many years (and many errors) was that people misinterpreted what he perceived to be his positive focus on excellence, and "limitless potential." At the conclusion of an assignment or event, when asked to provide his feedback, he would do so by providing positive observations, as well as a number of suggestions for potential improvement. While he thought he was simply supporting continuous quality improvement, he came to understand that those receiving the feedback took his responses to be an indication that he was unhappy or dissatisfied with their work. Worse yet, some feared they had failed his expectations.

Similarly, if someone asked for his input for an implementation, he often provided a list of umpteen things to consider. His intent was simply to offer advice to achieve excellence, but the input was received as overwhelming. The point being, Kyle was initially unaware that his strength sometimes had unintended, negative consequences.

Observation #4: The Humility–Ego Dichotomy

We typically place a high value on humility in our leaders [1]. In fact, if integrity is the attribute that often tops the list of "traits of effective leaders," humility is usually not too far behind. Our fourth observation is that successful leaders in academic medical centers understand and manifest an effective balance between humility and ego. This includes embracing their self-worth, understanding they are highly successful individuals, while simultaneously understanding and manifesting true (as opposed to disingenuous) humility.

If the concept of ego is a "person's sense of self-esteem or self-importance," [2] then we offer that it can be helpful (if not necessary) to have a *healthy, reasonable* dose. This may come as surprise, but leadership is not for the faint of heart. One's ego can be an advantageous partner when courage and decisiveness are needed, such as when making critical, time-sensitive decisions, managing challenging personalities, or leading up. And, if you think about it, who wants to be led by someone who does not believe in themselves or their vision? In sum, consider this thought from author Rick Warren, "True humility is not thinking less of yourself; it's thinking of yourself less." [3] The effective leader works not solely for their own benefit, but more importantly for the benefit of the organization and its members.

We have noted over our many years of observation and practice that "good" leaders share two important and related characteristics, two sides of the same "leadership coin." These characteristics create guard rails that help keep the leader's ego in check and provide the necessary balance between humility and ego. One side of the coin is *intellectual curiosity*, which we define as the desire to continually learn, grow, and stay fervently engaged. The leader with intellectual curiosity demonstrates and inspires continuous personal and organizational improvement. In this fashion, the leader remains open to exploration and discovery.

The other side of the coin is *intellectual humility*, the counterbalance to intellectual curiosity. No matter how much the leader learns, intellectual humility prevents them from ever thinking they have "arrived." Author and executive coach Jerry Colonna has a wonderful expression, "better humans make better leaders." [4] In our personal leadership journeys, we would say that the more we've learned and experienced, the less we feel we actually know. Humility allows for more curiosity.

The leaders who effectively manifest intellectual curiosity and humility also seem to share two other related traits we believe contribute significantly to their success, (1) creativity and (2) the ability to tolerate ambiguity. Creativity allows leaders to see issues differently, thereby framing problems in new ways. The result is a willingness to take appropriate risks, the development of novel solutions to problems, and the ability to guide others to accept and engage in these fresh solutions.[2]

---

[2] For more ideas about the use of creativity in leadership, check out the interview and podcast series with famous and well-established artists, "The Artist as Leader," from the Thomas S. Kenan Institute for the Arts at the University of North Carolina School of the Arts.

Next, effective leaders tolerate ambiguity. They understand that organizations are complex, that multiple interests and stakeholder views must be continuously taken into account, that emerging circumstances often alter a current course of action, and that problems or situations are more often than not, complex and multifactorial. Though this constant backdrop of ambiguity can be unsettling, and sometimes even demoralizing, effective leaders aren't deterred. Rather, they embrace the long view, recognizing that these issues are waves within a greater ocean. They don't worry themselves if it is high tide or low tide, they simply know, and are prepared for, the waves to keep coming.

Perhaps these traits are seen together in successful leaders because, oftentimes, creativity is the antidote to ambiguity. Staying generative and open to possibilities allows leaders to stay action-oriented and forward thinking. Even in the face of ambiguity they are able to maintain progress, examine situations with a fresh perspective, try different solutions, and gain more insights until an effective outcome or resolution is reached.

Observation #5: Reflective Is Effective

One of the quintessential practices of successful leaders is reflection, or purposeful and disciplined thinking and consideration. Based on the original work of Donald Schön, [5] three types of reflection have been described, including "reflection on action" which occurs *after* an event, "reflection in action" which occurs *during* an event, and "reflection for action" which occurs *before* a next or new event [6–8].

To acquire these skills of reflection, a new leader can begin by developing the habit to deliberately practice the art of "reflecting on" a given event. This includes reviewing the circumstances and outcomes, the leader's actions, the responses of others, and if/how the leader achieved their intended outcome. If it was not accomplished, then it is useful to consider how they might have done things differently to obtain a different outcome.

As the leader develops this reflective habit and begins to create generalizations from one event to the next, they will also find themselves becoming increasingly adept at "reflecting in" the moment. This skill involves the ability to think about what one is doing *while* they are doing it.[3] It is as if the leader is able to watch themselves in real-time and course correct to change their approach, tactics, course of action, etc., to improve the process, or outcome. It is the application of mindfulness.

If reflection "on" and "in" action becomes consistent and perhaps even an unconscious practice, the leader will naturally begin to adopt the skill of "reflection for action." A reflective leader learns from their experiences and applies lessons learned to the *next* situation, thus becoming increasingly more adept. They also gain the cumulative benefits of experience so as to avoid Reid Hoffman's observation that,

---

[3] This might be described has having an "out of body" experience, being able to watch oneself in action.

"for many people 'twenty years of experience' is really one year of experience repeated twenty times." [9].

Reflection influences self-improvement, impacting the powers of observation, inference, and decision-making. Reflection allows the leader to generalize what they learn from one event to another, providing the foundation for progressively more effective decision-making and actions. Adding this important resource to their armamentarium of competencies will serve the leader and the organization well.

Observation #6: The Value of Emotional Intelligence

In our observations, effective leaders almost always exhibit the set of skills, defined by Daniel Goleman as "emotional intelligence" or "EQ," [10] which include:

- Self-awareness
- Self-regulation
- Motivation
- Empathy
- Social skill

In general, leaders who are *self-aware* are realistic about their leadership capabilities. They readily recognize and understand their own strengths and areas for needed improvement. This allows them to be self-confident, while exhibiting the type of humility we described above. *Self-regulation* allows the leader to control their emotions and impulses, as well as to continually put events in perspective and manage their reactions. Effective leaders are *motivated* by the very work of leading, of setting a vision and making things better. They are patient, not easily discouraged and able to maintain a "long-view" as it pertains to the outcomes of their leadership.[4] We will speak to motivation more specifically in the next section.

Leaders in academic medical centers are very familiar with *empathy* as it pertains to patient care. The empathetic leader is similarly capable of considering others' needs and the potential impacts the leader's decisions have on them. Lastly, *social skills* reflect the compilation of communication and interpersonal skills and savvy that convey the leader's authenticity, especially in how they value the people they lead. Good relational skills facilitate team building and inspire high performance.

---

[4]As we noted above, effective leaders can tolerate ambiguity (as well as failure). Self-regulation and motivation are the attributes to facilitate this outcome.

Observation #7: The Compelling Motivation to Lead

Our final observation concerns a more detailed discussion of one of the elements of emotional intelligence, motivation. The concept of motivation essentially answers the question of *why* leaders lead. What draws them to do it and what keeps them engaged in good times and bad.

In the writings of Aurther Conan Doyle, detective Sherlock Holmes uses the expression, "the game is afoot." [11] The expression is similar to saying, "the pursuit is underway." While an odd expression today, in four simple words it encapsulates a leader's motivation perfectly. It clarifies both a call to action and an excitement of what is to come. It's like a rallying cry, expressing sheer joy at the opportunity to observe, be challenged, think, create, and act.

In another story, Holmes tells his colleague, Watson, "I play the game for the game's own sake." [12] Holmes savors his role, not necessarily for the outcome, but for the love of the process (although solving unsolvable crimes could hardly be considered trivial). And he just plain loves what he does. In our observation, one thing that seems evident of effective, engaged leaders is that they *love* to lead.

It's true that leaders can be motivated by many factors; the opportunity to realize their vision, to help the organization achieve its mission, to support others' career growth, or to shape culture, to name but a few important leadership responsibilities. Furthermore, a leader's decisions and direction are incredibly important and immensely consequential. They can literally change the course of history for people, organizations, communities, and countries. But despite these lofty motivations and weighty responsibilities, without true enjoyment for the work it is hard to be effective. People notice an unenthusiastic leader.

Contrary to being motivated by the love of leading, we have observed some leaders who are primarily motivated by being the "boss," seizing power, getting their way, or being recognized. Regrettably, this type of leader appears to be far more enamored with the title of leader than with the real work of leading. If your principal goal for becoming a leader is to be known or to have power, you will likely be disappointed with the leadership journey. We bring this to your attention because, as an emerging leader, you should know that leadership is seldom glamorous. It is hard work, and it is often lonely work. Put another way, when your motivation is to be recognized as important, you will seldom lead well. However, if your motivation is to lead well, others will recognize your importance.

How Do I Get Started?

Professional development for healthcare leaders is becoming more common-place in academic medical centers. Leadership development programs for emerging leaders are sprouting up, helping this population gain a better understanding of the art and science of good leadership. Executive and leadership coaching is also becoming increasingly commonplace, supporting the leader with their individual growth and development.[5]

There's no perfect leadership style. Each leader brings their own unique knowledge, skills, experiences, and values, along with assumptions, biases, and areas for needed improvement. Many academic medical centers offer strength and personality assessment instruments, helping the leader understand themselves more clearly. We've taken many such inventories[6] over the years, and have found each to offer valuable insights about our personality, traits, tendencies, etc. We encourage you to utilize these instruments to better understand your strengths and resultant tendencies. Spend time considering how your typical behavior changes when you are under more than the usual amount of stress, whether your behaviors manifest in the direction of your tendencies, and the impact this might have on your leadership effectiveness.

Consider how your strengths might be misinterpreted, misunderstood, or how they may, in fact, be counterproductive to your positive intent. Become familiar with your patterns of behavior on both good and bad days. Build this self-awareness to make more conscious choices about how to lead well, and how to course correct when necessary.

Coaching questions to ask yourself:

Recognize your intellectual curiosity and intellectual humility by considering how you would answer the following questions. While the questions may seem simple, the implications of your answers can have a far-reaching impact on your leadership success.

- Question 1: If you don't know something, are you brave enough to admit it and ask for help?
- Question 2: If you learn something new that is contrary to the position you currently hold, are you willing to change your mind?
- Question 3: If the situation calls for it, are you courageous enough to state, "I was wrong about that, and I'd like to learn more."?

---

[5] Check with your faculty development or human resources offices to see if they provide internal coaches, and/or have a list of recommended external providers.

[6] Popular tools we suggest you consider utilizing include the WorkPlace Big Five (WPB5), Myers-Briggs Type Indicator (MBTI), Herrmann Brain Dominance Instrument (HBDI), Enneagram, True Colors Personality Test, Gallup CliftonStrengths Assessment, and the Fundamental Interpersonal Relations Orientation and Behaviors (FIRO-B).

If your answer is "yes," to question 1, we submit you are demonstrating intellectual curiosity. A "yes" to question 2 is a demonstration of intellectual humility. And an answer of "yes" to question 3 offers evidence that you are demonstrating both intellectual curiosity and intellectual humility.

We propose that you revisit these small but powerful questions routinely throughout your leadership journey, and throughout your life.

Curious to learn more?

1. Colonna, J. (2019). Reboot: Leadership and the Art of Growing Up. Harper Business.
2. Epstein, R. (2018). Attending: Medicine, Mindfulness, and Humanity. Scribner Book Company.
3. Francis, S. L., & The Center for Courage & Renewal. (2018). The Courage Way: Leading and Living with Integrity. Berrett-Koehler Publishers.
4. Frankl, V. E. (2006). Man's Search for Meaning. Beacon Press.
5. Madden, C., & Kramer, R. (n.d.). Artist as Leader Conversations. Thomas S. Kenan Institute for the Arts; University of North Carolina School of the Arts. Retrieved April 2, 2022, from https://www.uncsa.edu/kenan/artist-as-leader/index.aspx
6. The Arbinger Institute. (2018). Leadership and Self-Deception: Getting Out of the Box. Berrett-Koehler Publishers.
7. Zander, R. S., & Zander, B. (2002). The Art of Possibility: Transforming Professional and Personal Life. Penguin Books.
8. HBR's 10 Must Reads on Emotional Intelligence. 2015. Boston, Harvard Business Review Press, Boston, MA.

References

1. Haden NK, Jenkins R. The 9 virtues of exceptional leaders: unlocking your leadership potential. Atlanta, GA: Deeds Publishing; 2015.
2. (n.d.). Oxford English Dictionary. Lexico; Oxford. Retrieved April 2, 2022, from https://www.
   lexico.com/en/definition/ego
3. Warren R. The purpose driven life: what on earth am I here for? Grand Rapids, MI: Zondervan
   Publishing; 2002.
4. Colonna J. Reboot: leadership and the art of growing up. New York, NY: HarperCollins; 2019.
5. Schön DA. The reflective practitioner: how professionals think in action. New York, NY: Basic
   Books, Inc.; 1983.
6. Olteanu C. Reflection-for-action and the choice or design of examples in the teaching of math-
   ematics. Math Ed Res J. 2017;29:349–67.
7. Killion J, Todnem G. A process of personal theory building. Educ Leadersh. 1991;48(6):14–7.
8. Grushka K, Hinde-McLeod J, Reynolds R. Reflecting upon reflection: theory and practice
   in one Australian university teacher education program. Reflective Pract. 2005;6(1):239–46.
9. Hoffman R. Twenty years of experience: a year of experience repeated twenty times. https://
   www.inspiware.com/twenty-years-of-experience
10. Goleman D. Emotional intelligence: why it can matter more than IQ. New York: Bantam
    Books; 1995.
11. Conan DA. The return of sherlock Holmes. New York, NY: W.R. Caldwell; 1905.
12. Conan DA. His last bow: some reminiscences of sherlock Holmes. United Kingdom: John
    Murray; 1917.

The Work of Leading in the Academic Medical Center

6

What Do Leaders Do?

In one scene of the cult classic movie, *Office Space* [1], two consultants meet with the various members of a company to better understand the work each does, ultimately for the purpose of deciding who should be let go. In a convoluted conversation with a customer service representative, one of the consultants finally asks, "What would ya' say you do here?"

If you aspire to lead, it seems logical that you should have a pretty good idea about what leaders do. But you might be surprised just how often this fundamental understanding is overlooked or not well understood, by both leaders and followers. When you make the transition to leadership (i.e., "administration"), you may even hear people say you've "gone over to the dark side." This is usually a humorous comment, but the underlying subtext suggests that some view administrators only as a "necessary evil."

Whether viewed as good, bad, or simply necessary, it is not uncommon for individuals to be placed in positions of leadership due to success in a related area. The new role is offered with the assumption that other (proxy) measures of success will translate in a broader leadership role. Take for example, the successful sports coach who is promoted to the role of athletic director, the successful salesperson who becomes regional manager, or in the case of the academic medical center, the successful researcher or clinician who is promoted to department chair.

We are not attempting with this chapter to present an exhaustive review of the purpose of leadership, but we will provide some insights into the question, "So, what would you say leaders do?" If you summarize the literature on what organizational leaders do, in general, you'll likely come up with a list somewhat like the following:

- Create and advance a compelling vision for the unit
- Develop and implement new initiatives (i.e., serve as a change agent)

© The Author(s), under exclusive license to Springer Nature Switzerland AG 2022
K. P. Meyer, R. Kramer, *Taking the Lead*,
https://doi.org/10.1007/978-3-031-16711-9_6

- Establish and promote an effective organizational culture
- Focus on the unit's strengths, results, and team building
- Manage crises
- Manage talent (i.e., recruit, develop, and advance personnel)
- Secure, align, and deploy resources (human, fiscal, capital, social, political, etc.)
- Set strategy and take deliberative risks to achieve the unit's mission

Each item on the list could be a chapter in and of itself (or a book, which is why there is a lot of published material on these topics). In reflecting on this list, we think the items represent the leader's *responsibilities,* but not necessarily the *purpose* of leadership. In other words, the list encapsulates the means or tools by which the leader gets things done. However, we propose there are three fundamental *purposes* of leadership: (1) creating meaning (to manage uncertainty), (2) developing people (and teams), and (3) balancing and aligning competing interests. Each of these purposes is addressed independently below, acknowledging they often overlap.

Leaders Create Meaning (and Manage Uncertainty)

Fundamentally, we think the vital, but often overlooked primary purpose of leadership is to *"create meaning."* To be clear, creating meaning is not an arbitrary fabrication of the leader's truth, engaging in revisionist history, or ascribing an interpretation of events in an effort to persuade or manipulate followers. Rather, we are suggesting that it is natural for members of the unit to look to the leader for a sense of understanding, stability, and security to help them interpret "environmental" events, and to gauge the overall "health" of the unit. Effective leaders communicate this sense of steadiness in their attitude, words, and actions every day (and even more so in difficult situations).

The leader's stabilizing force gives the unit purpose and mission focus by combating the universal nemesis that confronts all organizations, *uncertainty.* Uncertainty can arise from anywhere, from general environmental uncertainty to specific organizational uncertainty. Concerns about job security or reorganization, questions about the impact of new policies, proposed budget reductions, implications following a crisis, workload redistribution, getting a new supervisor, or implementing alternate work models are just a few examples in this latter category.

People usually do not do well in conditions of uncertainty [2]. It can significantly and negatively impact employee wellness, effectiveness, innovation, teamwork, satisfaction, productivity, engagement, and morale (the list could go on). Notably, uncertainty is also one of, if not the, primary barriers to change. And individuals with less tolerance for ambiguity are likely to struggle even more with uncertainty and change [3].

Consequently, one of the most important leadership responsibilities is managing uncertainty. We are purposeful in using the term "manage," as the leader cannot ever guarantee certainty, or ever really be in control of all aspects of the organization.

Leaders manage uncertainty by providing stability, which stems from creating (or ascribing) meaning to what might otherwise be considered ambiguous, random, or arbitrary events. In doing so they help the members of the unit interpret singular events, and also "connect the dots." By this we mean, the leader demonstrates how various events and outcomes impact or relate to the "big picture" vision and mission of the unit. Being purposeful, consistent, and transparent in communicating this message keeps individual members from creating inaccurate (often exaggerated) explanations about events or possible outcomes.

Take Another Look at the List

Noting this idea that the purpose of leadership is to create meaning, let's revisit the list of leadership responsibilities outlined above.

Leadership responsibility	How the leader creates meaning
Create and advance a compelling vision	*Defines where the unit is going, and how it will get there*
Develop and implement new initiatives (i.e., serve as a change agent)	*Defines how and why the unit needs to improve and progress*
Establish and promote an effective organizational culture	*Defines what the organization values, and how to interpret lived experiences in the unit*
Focus on the unit's strengths, results, and team building	*Defines team purpose and gives voice to the unit's employees*
Manage crises	*Defines unanticipated events and the unit's response, demonstrating the unit's resilience to these events*
Manage talent (i.e., recruit, develop, and advance personnel)	*Defines the alignment of employees' interests and abilities with the needs of the unit and provides opportunities for growth and advancement*
Secure, align, and deploy resources (human, fiscal, capital, social, political, etc.)	*Defines what the unit determines to be important and its importance to the organization*
Set strategy and take deliberative risks to achieve the unit's mission	*Defines why the unit exists and what it is intended to do*

From a *meaning making* perspective, at their core, these major leadership responsibilities help people understand the organization, its place in the world, and its value. As importantly, creating meaning allows the leader to guide the organization in dealing with the inevitable presence of ambiguity and uncertainty.

Developing People

One of the key barometers of whether you are both ready for, and will actually enjoy leadership, is whether you are excited to help others be successful. The point is that leadership is *not* about the leader. Rather, at its core, leadership is about providing the tools and resources people need to be successful, supporting their individual growth and advancement, as well as creating and environment for them to do great things collectively.[1] As the leader, you will need to embrace this quintessential purpose of leadership.

If you do, here's some good news—your emphasis on developing others will also very likely improve the unit's performance. Evidence strongly supports that the key to organizational success is employee engagement [4], a measure of the employee's emotional commitment to the organization. When considered from the perspective of the follower, the leader's job is to create the environment and culture that allows followers to thrive and succeed. A culture that facilitates engagement appreciates its employees, recognizes their contributions and accomplishments, and provides opportunities for growth and advancement.

We have seen that a healthy organizational culture comprises four fundamental elements, each of which can be established by the leader. The first is *purpose*. Certainly, the leader should know the members of their unit well enough that they can fully develop and maximally utilize each member's knowledge and skills by connecting each person's skills and attributes to the unit's overall mission. Furthermore, as it pertains to the team development, the leader creates the "culture of the collective." That is, the leader cultivates members' emotional connection to achieving something bigger than any one person could achieve on their own.

The second is a sense of *belonging*. That is, helping people be known and seen. People should have a voice within the organization, and the opportunity to actually influence outcomes and change.

Opportunities to promote *interpersonal engagement* is the third element. As humans, we value interaction and the opportunities to encourage and be supported. Not every employee will connect or "click" with everyone, but having workplace friendships is a strong inducement for engagement.

Lastly, we believe it's important to *have fun*. Humor is an invaluable resource. Granted, it can't always be fun, but if it's never enjoyable, work will get pretty dull, pretty fast.

So, through purpose, belonging, interpersonal engagement, and fun, the leader inspires their followers to do *great* things. This certainly makes for a compelling story, but is it reality? In the long run, yes, but it's probably not the day-to-day reality for most leaders (or followers, for that matter). By this we mean, great things don't typically happen every day. Rather, greatness is usually the culmination of persistent dedication to routine, repetitive, what might even be considered mundane, tasks. And the opposite effect is also true. Inaction seldom results in a disaster in the moment. But repeated inaction or lack of attention to a situation will ultimately catch up with the leader, and the unit. Often with disastrous results.

---

[1] Academic medical centers often distinguish between the employee positions of "faculty" and "staff." Development strategies and opportunities will likely be different for the members of these groups, but it's important to note that the leader is responsible for helping everyone in the unit develop and succeed.

George Washington Carver noted, "When you do the common things in life in an uncommon way, you will command the attention of the world." Hence, when it comes to developing people, we believe a key (and often overlooked) role of the leader is to ensure that effective and efficient policies, procedures, and structures are in place that expect, support, and reward, innovation, excellence, and accountability in the performance of "common things."

Unfortunately, in large bureaucracies like academic medical centers, policies and procedures can sometimes, inadvertently, promote inaction. It is the leader's responsibility to ensure that the unit's policies and procedures (hopefully the organization's as well), and the leader's decision-making, create a predisposition toward action. As Theodore Roosevelt noted, "In any moment of decision the best thing you can do is the right thing, the next best thing is the wrong thing, and the worst thing you can do is nothing." The leader models an action-orientation by focusing on what is attainable and within their control. The leader also encourages the members of their unit to be action-oriented by establishing a culture that invites creativity, supports reasonable risk-taking, and does not fear failure.

Lastly, we encourage leaders to use the means afforded them at the academic medical center to develop their people and support their teams. These include such things as nominating people (or teams) for awards, recognizing and promoting them, endorsing their involvement in national committees and professional governance structures, arranging for mentoring opportunities,[2] and supporting their leadership development and appointments for interim and permanent positions,[3] to name but a few. Supporting, championing, and developing followers will make the unit stronger, and the leadership journey immensely rewarding.

Balancing and Aligning Competing Interests

There are three sets of competing interests that are constantly at play within the academic medical center. While we describe them as "competing," they are not in and of themselves problematic, nor should the goal of the leader be to have one or more "win out" over the others. Rather, at various points in time, one or more of these interests will take precedence over the others. We explicitly define them here because we believe one of the primary responsibilities of academic medical center leaders is to manage, balance, and align these interests and their associated outcomes. Understanding them may also assist you in diagnosing problems that arise in your unit. The three sets of competing interests are:

---

[2] Mentoring opportunities can range from informal peer support to formal programming matching senior and junior faculty for one-on-one mentoring, to group mentoring (e.g., administrative colloquia, teaching academies, etc.).

[3] Strategies to develop and retain talent are part of succession planning, the purpose of which is both to identify and prepare individuals within the organization to assume specific key roles as vacancies become available. Effective succession planning complements recruitment of outside talent and can decrease the costs associated with talent searches, reduce the time needed for leadership transitions, and serve as a valuable tool for talent retention.

- Power versus Purpose
- Vision versus People
- Individual versus Collective

All three of these dichotomies overlap and intersect, but for the sake of our discussion, let's consider each separately.

Power Versus Purpose

As we have previously established, academic medical centers are large, bureaucratic organizations with multiple missions. Organizationally, they tend to exhibit more traditional, formal, hierarchical structures. This creates clearly identified units, individual roles and responsibilities, and alignment with the organization's overarching missions. Additionally, hierarchical models are also known for having a clearly delineated chain of command, more often than not identified by job title (e.g., Department Chair, Program Director, Dean, Nurse Manager, etc.).

As such, a leader can use the power of their position to get things done within the chain of command. Leadership expert John Maxwell [5] has identified five levels of leadership, the lowest being "position authority," which he indicates requires people to follow because they must. Granted, a leader does not want this to be their only source of authority, but it is none the less recognized and expected within the academic medical center. And for the emerging leader entering a formal leadership position, it may be their first source of power. Position authority affords the leader delegated permission to both direct others and to hold them accountable for the completion of their assigned activities. It also affords the bearer the right to pursue and accomplish the unit's purpose(s) through its people.

You have no doubt heard the adage written by British historian Lord Acton in the late nineteenth century, "absolute power corrupts absolutely." [6] Frequent reports about corrupt leaders continually reinforce our sense that power is inherently evil. Careful reflection on this adage, however, would suggest it is not power in and of itself that corrupts, rather how that power is exercised.

Herein lies the rub. Using power (authority) effectively to achieve the organization's purpose and support its people is its correct deployment. If the leader loses sight of the organization's purpose and its people, however, and their actions become more about themselves than those being led, power will corrupt. How do you know if this is happening? Well, there's no absolute diagnostic criteria, but here are a few things you might observe (in yourself or others) to alert you that power may be out of balance with purpose.

- The leader views themselves as central to the success of the organization and asserts that the organization would not succeed without their leadership.
- The leader ceases to acknowledge the value and work of others in the organization or blames people (often publicly) for any failures.

- The leader's communications focus increasingly on their role in the story.
- The leader insists on doing things "their way," even in the face of alternate recommendations or informed opposition.
- The leader stops seeking advice from their advisors (e.g., supervisor, Kitchen Cabinet).

In summary, there's a big problem looming on the horizon when power becomes about the leader's success as opposed to accomplishing the organization or unit's purpose.

Vision Versus People

Aligning the vision with the people who will carry it out is one of the most important aspects of leadership. Without a compelling, shared purpose and goals, an assembled group of people is more likely to either maintain the status quo or splinter among the self-interests of smaller subgroups. While subgroups may achieve some positive outcomes, it can be difficult to integrate the disparate outcomes and achieve a complete, preferred future.

On the other hand, the leader may create a compelling, innovative vision for the future, and yet their people do not believe it is achievable nor want to engage in seeing it come to fruition. Two questions arise for the leader's consideration: (1) Is it really a good vision (or the right vision for right now)? And (2) Do I have the right people to undertake the vision?

Regarding the first question, as an emerging leader it is important to build relationships with followers, but also to convey the vision for what the unit could become. Understand too that you don't just *present* a vision, you persuade people of the value of it. Expect, as an emerging leader, that not all your followers will immediately embrace your vision, especially if it represents a marked departure from business as usual. Since not everyone may be able to "see into the future," the new leader may need to do some coalition building, provide rationale and evidence, outline various scenarios, and engage their followers in collectively building a shared vision.

The difficulty in balancing vision and people is essentially the circumstance described by Jim Collins in examining how some companies become great [7]. Collins uses the metaphor of the company being a bus, and the leader being the bus driver. He notes that leaders of great companies *do not* begin by deciding where to drive the bus (the vision), but rather, they first discover who is on the bus. Leaders of great companies, Collins notes, "start by getting the right people on the bus, the wrong people off the bus, and the right people in the right seats." [8].

Individual Versus Collective

Every individual you lead will be different. They will have different attributes, skills, and points of view. And you should want that as a leader, as diversity of talent and thought improves decision making and innovation. To be an effective leader though, you will need to coalesce these diverse perspectives and talents to create a successful team, not just a group of assembled individuals.

An inherent challenge in this regard can be the promotion and tenure process used in most academic medical centers. These generally focus on individual achievement. Effective leaders who have both successful individuals and cohesive, supportive teams, often achieve this balance by establishing unit cultures that support collaboration, foster mentoring, promote team teaching and research, and celebrate the value of individual success for the good of the collective.

Individuals respond to success in different ways. We have seen individuals who are national or international "stars" in their respective fields lead large, successful teams as "first among equals," consistently acknowledging and promoting the value of the collective. Conversely, we have seen individuals who begin to quickly attribute the unit's success primarily to their contributions or believe that the unit exists solely to promote their own success.

Admittedly, academic medical centers are full of immensely talented, smart, super successful individuals. Their presence advances the reputation of the unit and the academic medical center, and can result in significant grant funding, assist in recruiting faculty and students, and of course, lead to important advancements and discoveries. Skillful leaders are deliberate in their communication and actions to promote and celebrate these individuals in a way that also celebrates and advances the collective. As NBA legend, six-time champion, and NBA Hall of Famer Michael Jordan said, "Talent wins games, but teamwork and intelligence win championships."

Sometimes a member of your unit may become progressively self-centered, perhaps generating resentment on the part of other members, or worse yet, causing the morale of the unit to decline. These situations rarely fix themselves, and if let go for a long time, can destroy a unit. So, we recommend you act sooner than later. Communicate your observations and concerns with the individual. Secure the assistance of a facilitator, if needed, for difficult conversations with the individual or the team, and consult with your human resources department. If change is not imminent, despite the individual's success you may decide that the healthiest long-term solution is to suggest the individual move on to another unit or institution that would be better able to support (or appreciate) their work.

To be clear, you want stars in your unit, but not at the expense of having a high performing team. The aim of leadership is to develop effective teams, where each member is recognized, valued, and celebrated for their unique contributions, where everyone embraces the collective goals of the unit and are recognized for its' achievements.

So… "What Would Ya' Say You Do Here?"

Our goal with this chapter was to provide you with some "philosophical" insights and encouragement about the leader's work. If creating meaning, facilitating the success of others, and inspiring your team to greatness is how you want to commit your time, then leadership is for you!

Periodic reflection will help you maintain your inspiration, perspective, and energy, especially when you might feel mired in the morass of managing day-to-day issues. Having a realistic understanding of the varied and sometimes competing interests expressed in the academic medical center will assist you in maintaining balance and alignment as you strive to both develop and advance individual members of your unit, as well as your entire team.

How Do I Get Started?

Formal leadership roles in the academic medical center are complex. The political landscape is varied and can be murky, egos can be large, and the competition very high. The emerging leader will do well to get as clear an understanding as possible on their new role, their span of control, the unit's financial health, the attributes and skills of their new workforce, and any other opportunities and landmines that can be surfaced. Getting the job is one thing but learning to be successful in the role is another.

Coaching questions to ask yourself:
- What did the person in this role prior to me do well and not so well?
- What does my new team need from me now, and what am I hearing we may need in the future?
- How do I learn who I can trust around me?
- How do I effectively hold space for dichotomies in this role and not be too quickly steered one way or another?
- What measures can I use to make sure I am on track and focused on the right things for this role and for this unit?
- How do I asses my skills at shaping and communicating meaning, and what can I do to get better at this skill?

Curious to learn more?

1. Arbinger Institute. (2015). Leadership and self-deception: Getting out of the box. San Francisco: Berrett-Koehler.
2. Rahim-Dillard, S. (2021, April 19). How Inclusive Is Your Leadership? Harvard Business Review; Harvard Business Review. https://hbr.org/2021/04/how-inclusive-is-your-leadership
3. Reynolds, A., & Lewis, D. (2018, April 2). Best Problem-Solving Teams. Harvard Business Review; Harvard Business Review. https://hbr.org/2018/04/the-two-traits-of-the-best-problem-solving-teams
4. Sanaghan, P., & Eberbach, K. (2013). The Seduction of the Leader. Academic Impressions. https://www.academicimpressions.com/product/seduction-leader/
5. Timms, M. (2016). Succession Planning that Works: The Critical Path of Leadership Development. Victoria, BC: Friesen Press.
6. Wooten, L. (n.d.). 5 Everyday Leadership Practices. President Wooten's Research; Simmons University. Retrieved January 17, 2022, from https://www.simmons.edu/about/university-leadership/president/research
7. Zackal, J. (2021, November 5). Handling the Strain of Being a Middle Manager. Higher Ed Jobs; Higher Ed Jobs. https://www.higheredjobs.com/articles/articleDisplay.cfm?ID = 2875

References

1. Judge M. (Director). Office Space (Film). Twentieth Century Fox 1999.
2. Pollard TM. Changes in mental well-being, blood pressure and total cholesterol levels during workplace reorganization: the impact of uncertainty. Work Stress. 2001;15(1):14–28. https://doi.org/10.1080/02678370110064609.
3. Steinhorst C. A leader's guide to managing employee uncertainty. Forbes. 2021. https://www.forbes.com/sites/curtsteinhorst/2021/06/16/a-leaders-guide-to-managing-employee-uncertainty/?sh=5a2fe26d9f11
4. Employee Engagement Statistics You Need to Know in 2021. January 4, 2021. https://blog.smarp.com/employee-engagement-8-statistics-you-need-to-know
5. Maxwell JC. The five levels of leadership: proven steps to maximize your potential. New York: Center Street; 2011.
6. Acton   Institute.   https://www.acton.org/pub/religion-liberty/volume-2-number-6/power-corrupts
7. Collins J. Good to great. Random House Business Books; 2001.
8. Collins J. 2001. Good to Great: Fast Company. https://www.jimcollins.com/article_topics/articles/good-to-great.html

Part II

Deciding About Decision-Making

The Multiple Dimensions of Decision-Making in the Academic Medical Center

7

A "Wide-Angle" View of Decision-Making

In academic medicine, thousands of decisions are made a day, from the routine to the complex, to the lifesaving. Leader's decisions span a range of areas including but not limited to, strategy, budget, personnel, recruitment, research, and operations. The cumulative impacts of the decisions made by leaders reverberate throughout the academic medical center. These impacts determine the experience a patient, student, or colleague has when they walk through the door, and ultimately determine the success (or failure) of the institution. And yet, the *process* of decision making is often an overlooked and taken for granted aspect of leadership.

Most leaders in academic medical centers come to the role having a background in clinical care, research, teaching, or a combination there of. We have observed these leaders are more prone to use a "diagnostic" approach to decision-making. By this, we mean the focus of decision-making is on the outcome or end product and not necessarily the process. Thus, as you enter your new leadership role, we suggest you take a step back to move beyond this one-dimensional approach to consider a more "wide-angle" view on the process of decision-making in an academic medical center.

Until people move into a leadership role, they may not think much about the factors that influence decisions or the implications that come from decisions. For the most part, people think the leader faces a decision, evaluates the facts, and makes a final determination. However, there are several implications and consequences that derive from not only *what* a decision is, but also why it is made, who gets to make it, when it is made, who learns of it first, where it is announced, and how it is communicated (including initially, as well as any secondary or follow-up communication utilized). You might think of these as political or constituent consequences.

These conditions are not unique to the academic medical center. They are present to some extent in all large, complex, bureaucratic organizations. As an emerging

K. P. Meyer, R. Kramer, *Taking the Lead*,
https://doi.org/10.1007/978-3-031-16711-9_7

leader, it is important that you understand and take into consideration these "meta" conditions surrounding your decision-making. By elevating your awareness, you will improve your capacity to understand decisions in a complex academic medical center, as well become a more effective decision-maker in your own right. Your understanding will also build your reputation as an effective and thoughtful leader, thereby enhancing your participation in the broader, institutional decision-making process. Perhaps you're familiar with the axiom, "if you're not at the table, you're likely on the menu." You want to be at the decision-making table!

Four Frames of Decision-Making

While it is beyond the scope of this book, the emerging leader would do well to gain familiarity with the concepts of organizational theory and organizational behavior. Briefly, organizational theory deals with how organizations function, and organizational behavior with how people within organizations function. Both fields influence decision-making.

- In our opinion, there are two outstanding books by Lee Bolman and Terrence Deal that masterfully summarize the literature on organizational theory and behavior, "Reframing Organizations: Artistry, Choice & Leadership," [1] and "How Great Leaders Think: The Art of Reframing." [2] We highly recommend both books. In their original work, Bolman and Deal introduce a simple but incredibly insightful conceptual model, that categorizes the literature into four ways of viewing an organization and its people. Bolman and Deal refer to these categories as "frames" or "lenses." The four frames are as follows:

- **Structural Frame:** Acknowledging the role of structure in determining organizational function, this frame focuses on such things as organizational charts, chain of command, standard operating procedures (SOPs), rules and regulations, work distribution, supervision, etc.
- **Human Resource Frame:** Acknowledging the value of the individuals in the organization, this frame focuses on such things as the emotional and psychological needs of employees, reward and recognition, relationships in the workplace, strategies to engage and empower employees, etc.
- **Political Frame:** Acknowledging that organizational resources are limited and those who control the resources strongly influence organizational performance and outcomes, this frame focuses on such things as power in organizational systems, conflict, competition for limited resources, advocacy, political shrewdness, etc.
- **Symbolic Frame:** Acknowledging that any decision or action can be interpreted by members of the organization to have a particular symbolic meaning (perhaps beyond its intent) this frame focuses on such things as organizational culture, rituals, ceremonies, stories, "heroes" of the organization, and their impact on creating meaning and inspiration for employees.

Bolman and Deal propose that the frames can assist the leader in thinking differently about a given situation or decision. In other words, the leader can "reframe" an issue to see it from a different perspective, thus gaining greater insight into the organization and its people, and thereby enhancing planning and decision-making. They state,

> How leaders think determines what they see, how they act, and what results they achieve. Each of the four lenses – structural, human resource, political, and symbolic – opens a new set of possibilities for leaders to use in finding their bearings and choosing a course [2]. (p. 20)

All the Frames, All the Time

Bolman and Deal offer that a given issue or problem might lend itself to being considered from a *particular* frame, and that changing the frame can also offer the leader new insights. We offer a slight variation, believing it is not only possible but also advisable to consider the implications of *all* four frames with *every* decision. In other words, decision-making can be enhanced if, as the leader, you are deliberate to engage in the *prospective* exercise of "looking through" all four frames simultaneously. This will help you both use your decision-making power to its maximum advantage and assist you in identifying the likely intended, and perhaps more importantly, *unintended* consequences of any given leadership decision.

The Nuances of Good Decision-Making

There are of course, different levels and complexities of decision-making. Major decisions typically take time to implement. Consider the time it takes to build a clinic, recruit and hire a new dean, or prepare a young medical student to become a great chief resident. Minor or immediate decisions may affect the circumstances of the present moment, such as a choice made during surgery, or engaging a colleague in a critical conversation.

Because the leader's decisions typically affect other people, it is important to consider the implications of a decision on a time continuum. In any occurrence, there are immediate and longer-term affects from your decisions.

You can also improve your decision-making ability by purposely reflecting on whether and how prior decisions (or consequences) might have created the circumstances affecting the decision you are currently contemplating (i.e., what happened before that got you where you are now with the situation?). Additionally, consider the immediate and longer-term consequences as your current decision "plays out" over time, remembering that the current decision may create conditions (good or bad) that will affect your next major decision.

This process is akin to coaching oneself. When making decisions, especially critical ones, explore multiple perspectives. Weight the practicality, the pros and cons of each. Consider the impact your decision will have on people and processes. How long will the decision take to achieve the desired outcome? And reflect on how the culture will respond to the decision.

If you consider each of the four frames described above, the intended and unintended consequences of any given decision relative to each frame, and examine those considerations over three time periods (past, present, future), you end up with a lot of data points for each decision! At first blush, this may seem an over burdensome approach, and perhaps not applicable to *every* decision. We believe however, with just a little practice, you will be surprised how adept you become at this process and the value it adds. It will become second nature, and the successful outcomes of your decision-making will prove the effectiveness of this approach.

Consider the following illustration: You assume the role of department chair of a rapidly expanding department. You determine rather quickly that the rapid expansion has led to a growth in clinical services, and consequently increased revenue. You also discover that because of the recent addition of several new members, departmental duties are not well delineated, resulting in some general operational inefficiencies.

To support the expansion of services and improve departmental efficiency, you decide to change the organizational chart by adding two new section chiefs and a staff administrator for each section. You confirm that increased clinic revenues will cover the costs of these changes. Additionally, you change the workload plan to enable better coverage for expanded clinics.

These seem like pretty straightforward "*structural*" frame changes. However, you would also be wise to capitalize on resulting message to the rest of the college that your department is successfully growing (*symbolic frame*). You may want to discuss with the dean that you will very likely need more resources in the not-too-distant future to continue your growth trajectory (*political frame*). Lastly, be aware that before you assign increased clinic coverage hours, consult with department members who will be affected by these changes. Without sufficient "run up" time to allow for adaptation, you may get some serious "push back" from disgruntled members of your department (*human resource frame*).

While the intent of your original decision was to facilitate expansion and improve efficiency, keep in mind that you may experience unintended consequences, such as resistance to change by members who think the department is growing too fast, or jealousy on the part of those who were not selected as new section chiefs. If you sense this might occur, it will behoove you to attempt to mitigate these outcomes with some behind the scenes conversations and negotiations prior to "going public" with your decisions.

Additionally, your decision will have the immediate impact of changing the departmental structure and increasing the number of clinics. However, if you reallocate resources toward this new structure and are not able to meet your projected revenue goals, you may be left with low departmental morale, and the inability to sustain the new structure over the long-term.

You can't predict every conceivable consequence of your decisions. The point is that you will be a more effective decision-maker and see greater success if you are purposeful in considering the various facets of your decisions *before* you make them. The goal is to gain greater clarity about the purpose of your decision and its likely outcome(s). In the example above, if you understood that a couple of already disgruntled department members will likely object to your decision, you might decide to move forward anyway, anticipating these members will move on. This potential outcome would then allow you to build a more collaborative and innovative culture. Anticipating results and scenarios will allow you to proactively manage the circumstances that follow your decision, illustrating that even seemingly "turbulent" outcomes might be purposeful and effective in the hands of a thoughtful decision-maker.

"Stay in Your Lane"

In your new role as leader, you will likely be invited to participate in decisions that affect the larger institution. As your knowledge, experience, and relationships in the organization grow, so likely will the invitations to participate in bigger and broader institutional decisions. As you find yourself in this situation, be practical. Remember, it will take time for you to prove yourself before your voice is heard and respected at the institutional level.

We mention this because emerging leaders can inadvertently get themselves into trouble early in their leadership journey as it pertains to their institutional role. A primary example is not understanding the scope of their decision-making. It probably goes without saying, but as an emerging leader you will have a limited span of control. In the early years of your leadership journey your decision-making autonomy will be "limited" to what is associated with your official position. You may meet some pushback, or worse yet, not be included in future decision-making processes if you choose to be too vocal in exceeding your scope. This can look like insisting you have the best answer to larger, institutional decisions while likely possessing limited leadership experience (i.e., credibility) and incomplete information.

To avoid the pitfalls associated with these circumstances, be deliberate about "staying in your lane." Make decisions pertaining to the things over which you have control or jurisdiction. This is not to say you cannot or should not contribute to institutional level decisions; just don't assume that because you are in your new role you have a *right* to be heard. At least in your early years of leadership, you may have greater success if you contribute when *invited* to do so.

If you believe you have a really good idea or perspective about a pending institutional decision and have not been invited to contribute, it might be the time to engage your supervisor with your idea. Your supervisor will likely have a larger span of control, and if they agree with your insight(s) they may be more successful than you to bring about the change. This approach may require some humility on your part, but it will increase the likelihood you are heard, and it will begin to establish your credibility as an effective problem solver.

How Do I Get Started?

Becoming adept at making good decisions is like building most any new skill – it takes time and practice. We have seen many emerging leaders who have good instincts, strong analytical skills, or are well trained and versed in models for decision making but fail to achieve the level of success they desire. It is through time, practice, occasional hard knocks, reflection, and continuous learning that the emerging leader develops consistently good decision-making skills that will ultimately become the foundation for their success.

Coaching questions to ask yourself:
- How can I get to the core of the issue that I am considering?
- What are the facts that may help inform my decision?
- Who will or may be impacted by my decision?
- What are *all* my options/choices I can consider (realistic and unrealistic)?
- What internal factors may be influencing my decision-making—my reasoning, my emotions, my instincts, my biases?
- Who have I seen make this type of decision before and handle it well? What did they choose to do and why?

Curious to learn more?
1. Ariely, Dan. 2010. Predictably Irrational, Revised and Expanded Edition: The Hidden Forces That Shape Our Decisions. New York City: Harper Perennial.
2. Bolman, Lee G. and Deal, Terrence E. 2013. Reframing Organizations: Artistry, Choice, and Leadership. San Francisco, CA: Jossey-Bass, a Wiley brand.
3. Bolman, Lee G., and Terrence E. Deal. 2014. How Great Leaders Think: The Art of Reframing. Hoboken, NJ: John Wiley & Sons Inc.
4. Friga, Paul N. "To Open or Not: Case Study in Strategic Decision-Making." Inside Higher Ed. Inside Higher Ed, August 14, 2020. https://www.insidehighered.com/views/2020/08/14/open-campuses-or-not-case-study-strategic-decision-making-opinion.
5. Heath, Chip, and Dan Heath. 2013. Decisive: How to Make Better Choices in Life and Work. Currency.
6. Kahneman, Daniel, 2011. Thinking, Fast and Slow. New York: Farrar, Straus and Giroux.

References

1. Bolman LG, Deal TE. Reframing organizations: artistry, choice, and leadership. San Francisco, CA: Jossey-Bass, a Wiley brand; 2013.
2. Bolman LG, Deal TE. How great leaders think: the art of reframing. Hoboken, NJ: John Wiley & Sons Inc; 2014.

Making Leadership Decisions Versus Clinical Decisions

8

We noted at the start that the purpose of this book is to provide insights to help you avoid some less recognized errors or pitfalls new leaders may experience in the academic medical center. Applying a familiar, and in many cases "automatic," *clinical* decision-making model to *administrative* decisions is one such area. New leaders who assume an administrative role in the academic medical center, having demonstrated success in the clinical mission, are particularly prone to this natural and often unintentional tendency.

In other words, it is not unusual to see clinicians (or researchers) turned leaders rely on the purpose and definition of decision-making that has been the source of their previous success. This is not to say that a clinical decision-making model is faulty or cannot be applied to solve administrative problems. However, without examining the impact of your decision-making model, you may inadvertently arrive at less than favorable outcomes.

When you move from a primary role as clinician or researcher to one of leader, the questions you are asked to address change. Thus, our caution to you as a new leader is that success in one avenue of work does not necessarily translate to success in another. Good technical skills are often very different from good leadership skills, as is the case with decision-making. Let's unpack this a bit by examining the general principles of health profession education[1].

What Are Health Professionals Taught?

Most health profession education programs are designed as structured or "lock-step" curricula, taught to a cohort of students. This design moves students through progressively more complex content as they learn the discipline-specific knowledge and competencies required to assume the role of the given health care professional.

---

[1] While we use the example of health professions education, this concept is equally applicable to the unique decision-making model of those educated as researchers.

K. P. Meyer, R. Kramer, *Taking the Lead*,
https://doi.org/10.1007/978-3-031-16711-9_8

Students learn the techniques for deriving, analyzing, and evaluating diagnostic data as it pertains to their profession, and then apply these skills in supervised clinical experiences. They are in essence learning to *think* like members of their chosen profession. In healthcare, we often refer to this thinking process as "clinical-decision making." As a general concept, "clinical decision making is a contextual, continuous, and evolving process, where data are gathered, interpreted, and evaluated in order to select an evidence-based choice of action." [1].

From our perspective, the key concept in this definition is "contextual." That is, every health profession has a different role and purpose in the healthcare system, and thus every healthcare professional will deploy their respective clinical decision-making model in the context of that unique role, gathering different data for different purposes, and having different choices of action that follow profession-specific methods of analyzing the data.

Take for example, physicians. They are trained to identify diagnostic clues relatively quickly that can help them derive a limited number of provisional (i.e., differential) diagnoses. They conduct tests or examinations, the results of which support or refute the potential diagnoses on this short list, in order to make a final diagnostic decision. Laboratory professionals on the other hand, are taught to make decisions with a focus on procedural order and accuracy. Quality control is the key factor in their decision-making and in the laboratory, there *is* one right answer. Physical therapists tend more toward decision-making models characterized by adaptability. They also conduct tests and make physical therapy diagnoses, selecting treatment approaches from an armamentarium of evidenced-based options. However, they may try different treatments or evolve the treatment based on the patient's response.

Why it Matters

The approaches above are of course generalizations, and no one approach is necessarily better than the others. They reflect the purpose of the profession, its academic roots, its historic training methods, and the healthcare delivery system in which the profession is practiced. All this to say, each profession has its own clinical decision-making model, and each professional is socialized through their initial training and subsequent experience to utilize (if not rely on) their model.

Consequently, when assuming a new leadership role, healthcare professionals may unintentionally, or even unconsciously, use their discipline specific *clinical* decision-making approach as their "default" *administrative* decision-making approach. The issue for *you* as a new leader is that the types of decisions you will need to make won't always lend themselves to your clinical decision-making model. Failing to recognize this and adapt your decision-making approach can lead to unnecessary leadership miscues simply due to your limited decision-making flexibility.

Take, for example, the new physician leader who employs a "diagnostic" decision-making model. When considering a leadership decision using this model, the focus is often on "diagnosing the problem." Consequently, when someone brings an issue to the new leader, their first question is likely, "What can I help you with?" Within seconds of hearing a little bit about the situation, the leader will consider two or three solutions and tell the individual what to do. Some people will be frustrated with this model, finding that it limits dialogue and exploration, and thus perceive it as too directive.

The new leader who comes from a laboratory background may believe there is one right answer to every administrative issue. As leader, they may not recognize the value of exploring multiple, equally plausible solutions to a problem, and thus be perceived by others as too rigid. Conversely, the former physical therapist turned leader, who was used to an adaptive and flexible approach to solving clinical problems, may now be perceived as too indecisive, unable to select a final declarative outcome from a series of equally acceptable choices. Lastly, consider a situation in which these three individuals are asked to make a collective leadership decision. It doesn't take much imagination to see how their different vantage points could contribute to difficulty in arriving at an agreed upon (not to mention effective) decision.

As clinicians gain expertise with their clinical decision-making model, they begin to listen for cues or key words, especially as they pertain to interviewing patients about symptoms or chief complaints. The idea of hearing one or two key words and then "filling in the gaps" is something we all do unconsciously, and in situations beyond just patient encounters. This helps us process information more quickly and efficiently, but it can also allow for unconscious bias or failing to see key data. Thus, after years of functioning in the academic medical center, you may enter your new leadership role thinking your clinician listening skills will serve you well as a leader.

Steven Sample and Rob Kramer (co-author of this book) in their respective books on leadership [2] and coaching [3] discuss the importance of leaders learning to listen well. Their definitions of listening are nuanced. Sample describes the skill of *"artful listening,"* [2] (italics added) noting that,

> The person who can turn listening into an art is one who goes beyond merely listening passively; he becomes intensely interested in what's being said and draws out the other person. In the process he gains not only additional details, but also valuable information on the filters and biases of the person presenting the information.[p.28]

Kramer notes that the components of *"conscious listening"* include a commitment to the value of listening (i.e., 'why bother'), setting asides one's own judgements, and seeking to understand the other's situation and perspective through curiosity and empathy [3].

As noted above, the overarching goal of the clinical decision-making process is to diagnose and determine a course of action, which can fuel a much more limited belief in, and reliance upon, listening (whether purposeful or inadvertent). In clinical practice, healthcare professionals get rewarded for thinking quickly, effectively, and accurately. In other words, for having answers. Given this mindset, listening in the ways described by Sample and Kramer can be a difficult task at best for a clinician turned leader. Moreover, *just* listening - without offering an "expert" answer or a direction - can seem a nearly impossible task. It is important for the new leader to become a great listener, and to also be purposeful in self-monitoring and not reverting to former habits and patterns.

A "Non-Decision" May Be the Best Decision

Healthcare is "action-oriented." In other words, people seek healthcare practitioners for help and answers. In fact, even the term we have been discussing, "clinical decision-*making*," demands that a decision "be made." While it may be true that the key responsibility of every healthcare professional is to do no harm, it is still expected that they *do something*.

Therefore, a leadership situation that can often be difficult for the new leader is the "no decision" decision. As Sample [2] notes, many leadership situations may not call for a response. In fact, the best response may be no response. We would add, at least not an *immediate* response. Take for example, the employee that comes to the leader with a complaint about a co-worker. There are no obvious legal, ethical, or moral concerns, rather the complainant "just" wants the leader to know the co-worker isn't working as hard as they should be (and if you think this example doesn't truly happen, think again).

What's the leader to do? Dismiss the complainant because their concern is irrelevant? Ask the complainant to come back after collecting data on the co-worker's work productivity? Commit to interviewing the co-worker to review their job responsibilities? Launch a time and motion study for the whole department to ensure equitable work distribution and output by all members?

The list could go on, but it is very likely that each choice on the list will come with some amount of disruption and high costs in time, effort, and emotional outlay. The best course of action to start? Listen to the complaint. Rather than being the expert and offering a solution, be curious, but non-committal. Ask pertinent and clarifying questions. As Sample notes, your artful listening will help you better understand the purpose, biases, and motives of the presenter. Let the person sharing be seen and fully heard. Acknowledge their concern and thank them for bringing it to your attention. To extend Kramer's thought, a commitment to the *value of listening* is also a demonstration of how much the leader *values the person* they are listening to.

Then "do nothing." While it may initially feel to you like inaction, you are actually employing "watchful waiting." This strategy (when appropriately utilized) can maintain relationships, prevent unnecessary work, allow time to gather further information, and generally improve decision-making. In some instances, problems may even solve themselves with just a little passage of time.

When Kyle (co-author of this book) first began his career in an academic medical center, one of his mentors told him very early on, "Never do anything until you've been asked three times." His mentor went on to explain, the first time you're asked to do something is generally by an overly zealous supervisor acting on an incomplete idea. The second time is usually because someone wants *you* to do *their* work. He concluded by saying that when you're asked a third time, "you know the boss means business."

There is of course some inherent risk in uniformly following this somewhat tongue-in-cheek advice, but over years of observation, we have found a kernel of truth in this facetious instruction, mostly in the form of recognizing that there are very few truly "emergency" leadership decisions that cannot be aptly considered over time. And perhaps more important, not every person or problem needs a decision—either from the leader, or at all. As you continue to develop your leadership skills, it is important that you learn there will be times when it may be better—for both you and the person(s) you are leading—to step away from your "diagnostic" role and just listen.

New Day, New Way

The combination of prior education and the professional responsibilities associated with working at an academic medical center can create some unique situations for emerging leaders that may not be readily apparent. As you enter your new leadership role, we recommend you think of it not simply as an extension of your former role(s), but as a completely different role, if not a completely different career.

We are proponents of the advice offered by executive coach and best-selling author Marshall Goldsmith in his book, "What Got You Here Won't Get You There." [4] This is not to suggest that the new leader's years of education and skill development in their field is of no value to their new role as leader. Rather, leadership is a different job than the "technical expert" of clinician, and it requires knowing and applying different behaviors and competencies. The good news is that leadership skills, just like clinical skills, can be learned. And as with clinical care, leadership expertise can be gained through intention, experience, reflection, learning, and practice.

How Do I Get Started?

Changing instincts that have been embedded through education and professional growth can be hard to adjust. However, a key to the leader's success lies in letting go of old habits and allowing space for new ones to be developed. Having a clear vision of "why" the change is needed is important.

First, take a step back to find your leadership "why." What drew you to take on a leadership role in the first place? Once you gain clarity on your why, then figure out how to make effective, appropriate decisions as a leader, and decipher how it differs from your skills as a clinician, scholar, or educator.

Next, if you haven't thought about how you make clinical decisions, below are some questions to guide you in elucidating the "unique" features of your professions' clinical decision-making approach:

- What is the primary intended outcome of a "typical" patient encounter from the perspective of your profession or specialty?
- What is the "typical" or "average" length of a patient encounter?
- Describe in 3–4 simple steps "how" you make clinical decisions.
- At what point in that process (if any) do you seek the input of others?
- What can result from you making an error in your decision process?

Coaching questions to ask yourself:
- How am I getting in my own way by relying on my clinical decision-making process?
- What do I need to adjust, or let go of all together?
- What can I hold on to that helps me in my leadership decision making?
- Who do I know that makes sound leadership decisions? What can I learn from them?
- What system can I put in place to catch myself and make needed adjustments when I notice the impulse to rely on old/unhelpful decision-making habits?
- What signals can I look out for to gauge the effectiveness of my leadership decision-making?

Curious to learn more?
1. Epstein, M.D., Ronald. 2017. Attending: Medicine, Mindfulness, and Humanity. New York: Scribner.
2. Frush, Benjamin W. 2021. "The "I Don't Know" Moment." Academic Medicine 96 (1): 67.
3. Khazan, Olga. 2014. "How Olympians Stay Motivated." The Atlantic. The Atlantic. February 7, 2014. https://www.theatlantic.com/health/archive/2014/02/how-olympians-stay-motivated/283643/.
4. Langer, Ellen J. 2000. "Mindful Learning." Current Directions in Psychological Science 9 (6): 220–23.

5. Ross, Philip E. 2006. "The Expert Mind." Scientific American 295 (2): 64–71.
6. Rotenstein, Lisa S., Robert S. Huckman, and Christine K. Cassel. 2021. "Making Doctors Effective Managers and Leaders: A Matter of Health and Well-Being." Academic Medicine 96 (5): 652–54.
7. Wright, Michael. [Michael Jr.]. 2015, September 10. *Know Your Why* [Video]. YouTube. https://www.youtube.com/watch?v=LZe5y2D60YU

References

1. Tiffen J, Corbridge SJ, Slimmer L. Enhancing clinical decision making: development of a contiguous definition and conceptual framework. J Prof Nurs. 2014;30(5):399–405.
2. Sample SB. The Contrarian's guide to leadership. San Francisco, CA: Jossey-Bass; 2002.
3. Kramer R. Stealth coaching: a roadmap to develop independent thinkers, proactive problem solvers, and exceptional leaders. 2nd ed. Eugene, OR: Luminare Press; 2020.
4. Goldsmith M, Reiter M. What got you here Won't get you there: how successful people become even more successful! New York, NY: Hyperion; 2007.

Getting Comfortable with the "Limits" of Decision-Making

9

We've talked a lot about strategies for improving your decision-making as a new leader, including raising awareness about the impact of a clinical decision-making model on your leadership decisions, as well as stepping back to consider a wide variety of implications related to your decisions. All this would seem to suggest we are advocating that the new leader adopt a more "extensive" decision making process. And we are. So, it may seem odd that we now turn to a discussion of accepting the *limits* of your decision-making.

We are highlighting the limits of decision making as a bit of a reality check. By this we mean that as leader, you will seldom have the luxury of fully investigating the parameters of a given decision and having the time and space to focus on one decision at a time. More likely, you will be in a rather constant state of juggling multiple issues and the array of decisions to go with them. The tendency of new leaders, given that you've had career success (and you'd like to keep it that way), is to "overthink" decisions, which can lead to frustration or delays on your part or on the part of those awaiting your decision.

Further, you will seldom make decisions in a vacuum. Others will influence or react to your decisions, and your decisions will evolve as you engage different stakeholders along a given decision-making trek. Making adaptations is valuable and necessary, as long as you don't find yourself endlessly second-guessing or "tweaking" your decisions ("paralysis by analysis"). For all these reasons, it is important to explicitly consider the realistic limits of decision-making.

The 70% Rule

The 70% Rule is a common notion in decision making, and often difficult for new leaders to accept. To start, consider it less of a "rule," and more of a good general guide, and try to let go of the expectation that you will, or can make perfect decisions.

The 70% Rule goes something like this: the leader will usually be able to gather or access about 70% of the information needed to make a *well-informed* decision in

K. P. Meyer, R. Kramer, *Taking the Lead*,
https://doi.org/10.1007/978-3-031-16711-9_9

a *reasonable* amount of time. Further, if acted upon, this 70% will *very likely* result in a good decision. In other words, 70% is generally a good enough start when it comes to leadership decision-making.

You may be asking yourself, "Why would you want to be *mostly* correct, when if you had 90% or more of the information, you could be even *more* correct? Here's why that is actually not a more effective approach:

- You will very likely never have 100% of the information you need, oftentimes not even 90%, so you may need to just accept that fact. Stated differently, there are never any guarantees when it comes to decision-making.
- Even if you could get another 10–20% of information it may not offer a sufficient improvement to the quality of the decision.
- Relatedly, the cost (yours or other's time, energy, and work) to get the additional 10–20% of information (assuming you could), may exceed the relative value of the information.
- Functioning under the 70% Rule keeps you from being the "bottle neck" on decisions, whether minor or major.
- Functioning under the 70% Rule sends a message to your leadership team that they too are free and encouraged to engage in deliberative and thoughtful risk taking as it pertains to decision-making.
- Functioning under the 70% Rule is what leaders do. Anyone can make a decision if they have 100% of the necessary information. But that is not *decision-making*, that is just the next step.

The trick to deploying this model effectively is to understand (or expand) your "reasonable risk tolerance" and to be able to increase both your patience with the decision-making process and your tolerance for ambiguity. Improving both takes deliberate practice and, admittedly, a bit of courage.

The 70% Rule's Impact on Change

As we discuss in greater detail in Chap. 16, one of the primary functions of the leader is to serve as a change agent. We have found the 70% Rule to also be an effective conceptual guide for change, and base this on the work of Everett Rogers [1, 2], who proposed a theory explaining how new ideas and technologies are adopted, including a description of five types of "adopters". We believe Roger's theory and the 70% Rule can be combined to consider how a leader might promote a new change (see Fig. 9.1).

To illustrate, consider Roger's depiction of the five types of adopters (each in capital letters) distributed on a bell-shaped curve (Fig. 9.1). The leader (along with other "innovators" in the unit) will likely be joined by the "early adopters" in a given change initiative (assuming the change is rationale and productive). Rogers notes that "early adopters" are influential, and often highly regarded, so their acceptance of a change initiative will be observed by members of the "early

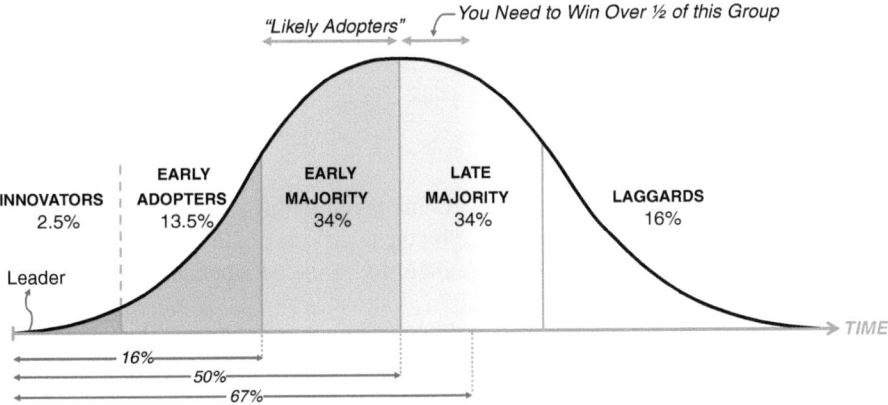

Fig. 9.1 70% rule applied to change management

majority," who although more risk averse will value the decisions of the "early adopters." Consequently, in introducing a change initiative, a leader could fairly readily achieve a 50% level of support within the unit. What we like about using the 70% Rule along with the Roger's model, is it suggests that the leader can likely ensure the adoption of change with approximately two-thirds support, and not 90–100%. Thus, to reach a two-thirds majority, the leader will need to secure the support from one-half of the "late majority." More is to come, below, on how to enroll the "late majority."

These of course are generalizations, and not every member of the unit will fit neatly into one of the "adopter" categories. It won't take long for you to determine however, which members of your unit at least fit "loosely" in the categories. The other reason we like this approach is that it identifies the value in having a different and deliberate strategy for each group to achieve a two-thirds majority. Of note, in our view it is ineffective for the leader to spend much time or energy on the 16% of "laggards" who will be the last to adopt (if ever) change.

As leader, we consider you an "innovator." But innovators exist at all levels, so don't overlook the opportunity to enroll other informal leaders on your team in this role, as well. In most instances, the small group of "innovators" will soon be joined by the members of your executive team or cabinet to make up the "early adopters" group that will help lead your change initiative.

Be sure this group is aligned with you regarding the change initiative. Expressly invite them to adopt the change and extol its benefits to the "early majority." Develop communication strategies that identify the rationale and intended positive outcomes of the change initiative, and personalize the value of the proposed change, ensuring you address any concerns that could be raised by the "early majority."

Member of the "early adopters" and "early majority" need to be genuine and consistent in their communication with other members of the unit, especially with the very important "late majority," some of whom will need to be won over to help you reach the magic two-thirds number.

The "Late Majority"

In general, members of the "late majority" are less tolerant to ambiguity, more skeptical and risk averse, and less influenced by the decisions of the "early adopters" and "early majority." Members of the "late majority" may be amenable to change, but they will need more proof, as well as more assurances about, "what will happen if it doesn't work?" To secure sufficient influential data demonstrating the value of the proposed change, you may need to utilize some trial balloons or do some pilot testing. But be assured, members of the "late majority" will be observing the "early adopters" and "early majority," so assuming results are positive, the data alone may be sufficient to gain their support. It may also be helpful to have a sufficient timeline for the full adoption of change, providing members of the "late majority" time to adapt.

Remember, you only need to gain the support of one-half of "late adopters" to achieve the 70% Rule. And convincing the additional 17% of the "late majority" that change is necessary (or beneficial) may require considerable time and effort that will likely not alter the outcome. Be cautious, however, with this half of the "late majority." Disregarding their needs or not attempting to address their concerns may, at best, have them join the "laggards," and at worst become active resistors to current or future change initiatives.

Being Deliberate about Deliberative Decision-Making

We've tried to establish the importance of employing both an effective and reflective decision-making process, while acknowledging the limitations in time and human capacity that confront even the best leaders. So, if the most a leader can hope for is to obtain 70% of the information needed to make a decision, how do you ensure you obtain the 'most helpful' 70%?

One strategy we recommend is to understand and employ the concept of "deliberative" decision-making. This is not to be confused with being thoughtful and careful (i.e., "deliberate" decision-making), although we advocate for that, too. To really understand deliberative decision-making, you might contrast it with how decisions are often made in the academic medical center (and most places for that matter).

It is typical, perhaps even expected, that stakeholders involved in a decision-making process view the issues of the decision through their *own* lenses and biases, whether conscious or unconscious. These lenses are a compilation of the decision-makers' role, experiences, values, relationships, and expectations, and in many instances result in a *pre-determined* outcome or "position" on the part of each decision-maker. "Positions" can be purposeful or unconscious, but regardless, they prevent the holder from seeing other alternatives. Consequently, some individuals may be deeply entrenched in their positions, and no amount of data or negotiation could change their mind.

A group of individuals with unalterable positions will not generate the most helpful 70% decision making data. In such a case, the decision makers may not be able to reach a decision, or they reach an unhelpful consensus decision. Consensus in this case is a euphemism for each stakeholder making some small concession at the margin of their position to reach a decision that more or less maintains the status quo. In other words, a collective group of decision-makers unwilling to move from their positions is a recipe for poor decision-making.

To combat this outcome, consider applying the characteristics of a "deliberative" decision making process, as legal scholar Cass Sunstein [3] considers for effective self-governance. In this process, decision-makers engage in a collective dialogue *for the express purpose* of scrutinizing positions and proposed outcomes, not just espousing positions.

For this collective evaluation process to work, however, two key elements must exist. The first is obtaining each participants' willingness and ability to *purposefully* distance themselves from their own positions in order to engage in the evaluation process. The second, which is perhaps even more difficult, is a willingness by each participant to commit to *revising* their position as the collective discussion yields new information and alternative perspectives.

This process may be hard to implement and even harder to consistently adhere to. Perhaps because it is contrary to contemporary public discourse's influence that people need to strongly adhere to their positions. However, the goal is to create an atmosphere for safe, open dialogue and debate that invites and values a wide variety of diverse thoughts, giving equal voice to every opinion or position. We believe this process can be reached by consistently implementing ground rules for deliberative decision-making, and we have seen the result be more effective, sustainable, and widely accepted decisions.

How Do I Get Started?

Hopefully you are starting to see that effective decision-making can be a complex and nuanced practice. Adding tools to your decision-making toolbox is far easier than knowing the limits and full use of those tools. By understanding the boundaries of decision-making, the leader has more clarity on which way to proceed, who to engage in the process, and what tools to specifically use for various situations.

Coaching questions to ask yourself:
- How willing am I to do the work needed to get the needed majority of people on board with a change initiative?
- Who do I see as my biggest champions in this situation and how will I partner with them?
- What do my potential "early adopters" and "early majority" need to get on board with a proposed change?
- How will I mitigate the critics so as not to distract others from the goal?
- How can I begin to implement a deliberative decision-making culture and process?
- What strategies can I employ to ensure open dialogue? How can I restrain those who speak too much and encourage those who speak too infrequently?
- If not me, who is the best person(s) to guide deliberative decision-making conversations?
- What aspects of this process are in my control, and what parts do I need to accept?

Curious to learn more?
1. Cialdini, R. B. (1993). Influence: Science and practice. New York: HarperCollins College Publishers.
2. Covey, S. R. (2004). The 7 habits of highly effective people: Restoring the character ethic ([Rev. ed.].). Free Press.
3. Grenny, J. (2013). Influencer: The new science of leading change. New York: McGraw-Hill.
4. Schein, E. H. (1998). Process consultation: Vol. 1. Reading, MA: Addison-Wesley.

References

1. Rogers EM. Diffusion of innovations. New York: Free Press of Glencoe; 1962.
2. Understanding early adopters and customer adoption patterns. Interaction Design Foundation. https://www.interaction-design.org/literature/article/understanding-early-adopters-and-customer-adoption-patterns
3. Sunstein CR. Beyond the republican revival. Yale Law J. 1988;97(1539):1539–90.

Decisions about Your Academic Medical Center Career Trajectory

10

Developing Your Career as Leader

In the last three chapters, we have examined a number of considerations about decision-making, with the goal of providing you a broader understanding about its characteristics. We have discussed the multiple dimensions of decisions, the impact of your clinical decision-making model on your leadership decisions, and the limits of decision-making. In this chapter we "turn inward," providing guidance on how you might consider decisions regarding your career development and trajectory as a leader.

New leaders are equipped with energy, great intentions, and abundant enthusiasm. As such, there is a phenomenon that occurs with some degree of regularity for emerging leaders in academic medical centers—the relentless presence of "opportunities" to develop and exercise leadership skills. This is especially noticeable when new leaders demonstrate early success and promise. Thus, the situation new leaders grapple with is deciding which of these opportunities to pursue. Additionally (and a word of caution), the term "opportunity" conveys the idea most of us will recognize in the often-heard statement, "Have I got an opportunity for you."

Opportunities Abound

There are multiple reasons that opportunities are so prevalent within academic medical centers. A primary one being that these institutions are by their very nature places where ideas are generated, and where members value altruism. As we noted earlier, academic medical centers represent a "loosely coupled" organizational structure, involving multiple interdependent units that act somewhat autonomously and with limited coordination. The result is a multitude of ideas continually springing up from everywhere. These ideas are often not "formal," in that they do not

© The Author(s), under exclusive license to Springer Nature Switzerland AG 2022
K. P. Meyer, R. Kramer, *Taking the Lead*,
https://doi.org/10.1007/978-3-031-16711-9_10

necessarily carry a requirement for completion, and they may not be supported by a budget allocation. Thus, the purveyor of the idea often seeks collaborative partners to pursue the opportunity.

A third common source of opportunities are the professional organizations and associations that provide oversight, guidance, advocacy, and general support of the various professions within academic medical centers. Most if not all of these professions are "self-governing." As a result, endless volunteer leadership opportunities exist to serve in governance roles and give back to one's profession. This type of professional service is also highly valued and supported by the academic medical center, as it is often considered an important element for promotion and tenure.

Effective leadership is essential in the above examples, as each involves shepherding numerous people across multiple units (or organizations) to voluntarily contribute time and talent (and in some instances, financial resources) to bring ideas and initiatives to their full realization and implementation. They require the skills of assembling members, building coalitions and consensus, maintaining timelines, managing group conflict, and being accountable to complete the task. And as is often the case, emerging leaders have the eagerness and energy to serve.

Abundance Restraint

The common problem with an abundance of opportunities for the emerging leader is being inclined to say "yes," more often than "no." As others across the organization, and across the country, begin to notice the emerging leader's successes and growing reputation, an increasing number of opportunities will arise. The features of these new opportunities, combined with professional altruism and increased achievements, can create an emerging leader's false belief that taking on all these opportunities is necessary to maintain their current trajectory of success.

The unfortunate yet common result of this deluge of abundance is the new leader feeling overwhelmed by more opportunities than they could ever hope to manage. A paradox of sorts emerges over time. The new leader takes on more, they experience a splintering of their attention and effort, their performance decreases, and concern over their reputation and/or abilities arises. To combat this, the emerging leader may try increasing their work volume and hours. Unfortunately, they'll soon find themselves stuck on a treadmill, often at the expense of their primary responsibilities—main job, health, personal life, or some combination of them all. So, for the emerging leader's long-term success, both professionally and in maintaining good health and well-being, we offer that you need to learn when to say "yes," and when to say "no." Also, since saying "no" is sometimes difficult, how to say "no" is an important and artful skill to develop.

When Your Supervisor Speaks, Listen

To not overcommit yourself, it is important to distinguish opportunities you "could" do from what you "should" do. We say this because sometimes a supervisor or other senior leader may present you with an opportunity or invitation to participate in an initiative. It probably goes without saying, but what may come in the form of an "invitation" should almost always be understood as a "polite directive." In describing this situation, people sometimes say they've been "voluntold" to participate. Obviously, it's not in your best interest to say "no" to these types of opportunities.

The good news is that when your supervisor or other senior leader steers you towards opportunities for leadership development, they likely know your personal interests and are explicitly engaging you to achieve some intended growth outcomes. For example, suppose you are a division chief in a college of medicine who aspires to one day be a department chair. The dean of the college may ask you to chair a search committee for another department's open chair position. This opportunity would afford you the experience of managing a search committee and allow you to learn first-hand the requisite attributes necessary to be a department chair. Though it is politically smart to say "yes" to this opportunity, it is also clearly a chance the dean is giving you to (1) further demonstrate your leadership skills with colleagues you might not otherwise engage, and (2) position you better for future chair opportunities.

Keep a look out for these opportunities as they come your way. For example:

- The education program director in the college of allied health professions wants to expand his knowledge and scope as an expert educator. He is asked by the vice-chancellor of academic affairs to sit on a special task force to develop a campus-based e-Learning Center.
- A senior faculty member aspires to one day assume a formal leadership position. The chair of her department suggests she run for election to serve on the Faculty Senate and offers to provide her protected time if elected.

These opportunities represent clear, deliberate, formal experiences designed to further the emerging leader's development and to demonstrate their competence to a wider audience, and almost always necessitate a "yes."

As noted above however, the emerging leader will also be presented with numerous opportunities for which they have more latitude to say "no." There are countless examples of these activities: standing committees, ad hoc committees for the development of any number of policies and procedures, curriculum revision groups, program evaluation committees, professional and community boards. The list goes on and on… and on. It is wise to thoughtfully consider these opportunities before responding. If useful, talk to a mentor, supervisor, or trusted colleague for their perspective. There may be nothing wrong with having an initial predisposition to say "no, thank you," or "not right now."

Strategies for Picking the "Right" Opportunities

How should the emerging leader pick the "right" opportunities? We recognize that the conditions that surround a "yes," or a "no" decision are as innumerable as the opportunities themselves, and the same conditions may result in a different answer at different times. With this in mind, there are a few strategies we believe will assist you in saying "yes" to the "right" opportunities (and "no" to those that may not be in your best interest).

For starters, having clarity about your personal, professional, and organization's mission and vision is critical. Be deliberate about identifying the goals you have for the unit you lead, and for your own professional development. Doing so will help you maintain focus in decision-making. You can evaluate any given opportunity from the perspective of both how well it aligns with your own mission and vision, and whether it will help to achieve your and your organization's desired outcomes.

It's true that life in an academic medical center is all about participating in multiple activities. Some participation is necessary, but it's easy to find yourself on too many committees, leading too many initiatives, or being involved with too many professional organizations. Remain cognizant about meeting the expectations for promotion and tenure. Familiarize yourself with the promotion and tenure guidelines and productivity expectations, as they may offer useful guidance for evaluating whether to say "yes" or "no" to opportunities.

Women and persons from underrepresented groups are particularly susceptible to the phenomena of having service activities limit their capacity to meet other productivity standards for timely promotion. They may be asked to participate (or feel obligated to volunteer) [1] on multiple committees or in numerous initiatives, representing a certain group(s) or perceived point of view. The institutional goal of being inclusive can (and often does) place an undue burden of responsibility on these individuals. And though the invitation's intent may be good, it can be an overwhelming responsibility for the invitee. The resulting stress and burnout can limit the individual's capacity to demonstrate the teaching, research, clinical care, and/or administrative productivity needed to achieve promotion and advance their career [2].

Thus, as any new opportunity is presented to you, we encourage you to ask yourself if the opportunity aligns not only with your goals but also with your strengths. Conversely, an opportunity may present a reasonable opportunity for you to work on something you need to improve. Find out why you are being invited to participate in the opportunity, why the inviter thinks you are the right person, as well as why they think you will be able to succeed in the role. Ambiguous answers such as, "Because I know you'll get the job done," or "I just feel like you're the right person to lead this initiative," are insufficient and may be a good clue to say "no" to the opportunity.

If, however, you think the opportunity could help you develop and expand your skills, make sure your developmental goal is clearly identified and mutually agreed upon. Additionally, do not hesitate to gather clear expectations and the inviter's commitment to offer appropriate support, as necessary.

Keep in mind that sometimes opportunities will present that may not fully align with your developmental goals or availability. Yet it may still be in your best interest (i.e., the politically smart thing to do) to say "yes." Evaluating these types of opportunities requires some political savvy. Some reasons you may want to say "yes" would include, (1) the benefit to your reputation, (2) gaining early exposure as an effective leader, (2) the desire to support a colleague, program, or unit, (3) a chance to build a valuable relationship, (4) creating a foundation for future opportunities, or (5) you possess a unique skill that is necessary for the success of the initiative.

If you do say "yes" to an ill-timed opportunity, it can be helpful to clearly identify your role and function, verify the measures for success, and determine your timeline for participation. Being explicit about these conditions will allow you to participate in the initiative, retain some degree of control pertaining to your engagement, and potentially allow you to "step out" when your duties are completed.

A good relationship with your immediate supervisor can be immensely helpful in determining when to say "yes" or "no" to an opportunity. Make sure to have periodic discussions with your supervisor about your goals and activities. Be as specific as possible about your aspirations, the substantiating rationale, and your plans and timeline for promotion (and tenure). Seek your supervisor's input so you and they arrive at "mutually determined" goals. With a clear plan in place for your continued development, you may then take any new opportunity to your supervisor for their opinion. If you or they do not think the opportunity is in your best interest, it allows you to say "no" with the support of your supervisor. Note: If you do not have a strong relationship with your supervisor, it would be useful to find a mentor or other colleague who can help funnel opportunities your way, as well as help you think through when to say "yes" or "no," and the implications of either decision.

A Model for Evaluating Opportunities in the AMC

A good analogy that is especially pertinent within an academic medical center is to consider an opportunity as you would a new research project. At the outset of a collaborative research project, you might ask your proposed research collaborator(s) a series of questions to clarify the process and outcome(s). These questions could include:

- What is the goal of the project? (i.e., how does it also advance my areas of interests, skills, or vision?)
- What resources do we have at our disposal?
- Who is responsible to do what? (i.e., clarify your role)
- How long do we anticipate the project will take?
- How will we know when we are done?
- How will we measure success?
- Who will be first author on the manuscript (i.e., How will we communicate our work on the project and who will get credit?)

We believe it is your prerogative to ask the inviter these types of questions from a place of curiosity, including follow up questions such as "tell me more?" and "what would that look like?", to thoughtfully obtain the information and clarity you need. If the inviter's responses are vague, or they cannot or will not answer these questions, it might be the evidence you need to say "no" to the opportunity.

Committing to Opportunities

As a final thought on selecting opportunities, we encourage you to fully commit to your "yesses" and "no's." If you agree to an opportunity, make sure you go all in. The goal of a "yes" opportunity is to develop your skills and your career. Saying "yes" and doing a mediocre job is worse than just saying "no" at the outset. On the other hand, offhandedly saying "no" to every opportunity is a surefire way to eliminate any future opportunities. We encourage you to put careful thought and consideration into the opportunity before declining. If your "no" is definitive, be prepared to explain your process for considering the invitation, the rationale for declining, and thank the inviter for the opportunity. Lastly, if you are so inclined, invite them to ask you again at a time that might be better. If you do so, however, be prepared to say "yes" the next time the opportunity arises.

There is also additional data we recommend you attend to after you say "no." The inviter's response will likely give insight into their motive for presenting the opportunity in the first place. People truly interested in your development may express disappointment in your decision but will generally acknowledge your rationale, and often commit to asking again. Those who wanted a "yes" from you so they could get the initiative off their own desk are seldom interested in this conversation, as with your "no" they are already moving on to ask the next person.

Concluding Thoughts

The academic medical center abounds in ideas and opportunities to develop your leadership skills. There will be more opportunities and work than you will ever be able to accomplish. However, with proper mentorship and guidance we believe you can capitalize on these opportunities to have a remarkable leadership career. The key is knowing when to say "yes," and when to say "no," and committing to your decision. Opportunities often present themselves in a random fashion. Having an overarching plan to guide your unit and your leadership development will keep you focused on participating in the "right" opportunities.

The famous investor Warren Buffett said, "The difference between successful people and really successful people is that really successful people say no to almost everything." While we are not advocating you say "no" to almost everything, we do believe the optimal outcome for emerging leaders is to make selective "yes" decisions on opportunities that align your skills, passions, and altruism with promotion and tenure (and other) advancement goals and expectations. This will allow you to make significant contributions to the growth and improvement of the institution while also ensuring you meet your own individual advancement goals.

How Do I Get Started?

The fundamental career issue confronting most high performing emerging leaders is to find their balance in work opportunities. The myriad of prospects can be career enhancers or career derailers. Be thoughtful and strategic in assessing each opportunity that comes your way.

Coaching questions to ask yourself:
- Does this opportunity sound interesting to me? Why or why not?
- How will my participation in this opportunity get me where I want to go?
- Is it politically savvy to say "yes" (or "no") to this opportunity?
- What does my gut tell me about this invitation?
- If I say "yes" to this invitation, what do I need to offload or shift to effectively participate?
- After participating in any opportunity, ask yourself: was that worth it; and specifically, why or why not? Use this accumulating "data set" to help guide your next career decision.

Curious to learn more?
1. Bach, B. (2016, March 23). 5 Questions: Sabine Girod on gender leadership bias in academic medicine. Stanford Medicine News Center; Stanford School of Medicine. https://med.stanford.edu/news/all-news/2016/03/sabine-girod-on-gender-leadership-bias-in-academic-medicine.html
2. Godbee, B. (2018, May 14). Making Career Moves by Saying No. Inside Higher Ed. https://www.insidehighered.com/advice/2018/05/14/why-its-positive-thing-say-no-your-career-opinion
3. Sklar, David P. MD Leadership in Academic Medicine: Purpose, People, and Programs, Academic Medicine: February 2018 - Volume 93 - Issue 2 - p 145–148. doi: 10.1097/ACM.0000000000002048
4. Vaillancourt, A. M. (2013, September 3). Are You Disappointing the Right People? The Chronicle of Higher Education. https://www.chronicle.com/blogs/onhiring/are-you-disappointing-the-right-people?cid2=gen_login_refresh&cid=gen_sign_in
5. Zambrana, R. E. (2018). Toxic Ivory Towers: The Consequences of Work Stress on Underrepresented Minority Faculty. Rutgers University Press.

References

1. Armijo PR, Silver JK, Larson AR, Asante P, Shillcutt S. Citizenship tasks and women physicians: additional woman tax in academic medicine? J Womens Health (Larchmt). 2021;30(7):935–43. https://doi.org/10.1089/jwh.2020.8482. Epub 2020 Nov 17
2. Zambrana RE. Toxic ivory towers: the consequences of work stress on underrepresented minority faculty. Rutgers University Press; 2018.

Part III

It's the Little (or Not So Little) Things

Leading by Following

11

A mentor of co-author, Kyle, summarized the entire concept of leadership in a single sentence when he said, "If you want to know if you're a leader, turn around." We've found this advice to be true. One's ability to lead depends on the willingness of others to follow. For many new leaders in the academic medical center, however, the most underappreciated part of assuming a leadership role isn't learning to lead well, but rather, learning to follow well. We believe that good followership is foundational to good leadership.

In this chapter we'll examine numerous aspects for leaders learning to be good followers. These include following their supervisor(s), those they lead, and other leaders. Our goal is to assist new leaders in becoming astute followers, ultimately enhancing their leadership success.

Following Your Supervisor(s): Tending to Their Tendencies

We've established that academic medical centers consist of loosely coupled, often matrixed units, each with their own unit-based structure and culture, collectively assembled within an overarching organization-wide hierarchy. As a result, the academic and research components of a unit typically report up through vice-chancellors on the academic side of the house, and the clinical components typically report up through the health system. This is a complicated way of saying that in academic medical centers, "every boss has a boss," and many times more than one.

In assuming a formal leadership role, the organization's hierarchy becomes much more real, and the new leader quickly learns that any leadership autonomy is *granted* rather than assumed. New leaders need to earn the respect of their superiors to gain or maintain autonomy. Such delegated authority provides the leader space to make decisions, to make reasonable mistakes, to control and direct resources, and to create and realize a strategic vision for their unit.

We believe there is far more to following your supervisor(s) than just doing what you're told to do. Leaders who "follow well" and develop effective reciprocal relationships with their supervisor(s) learn how to anticipate and meet their needs. Even if they don't express it, most leaders of other leaders hold to the adage, "Help me help you."[1]

And in general, the new leader understands their job is to help the people they report to be successful. Thus, leaders who follow well ensure each of their supervisor(s) is well-informed with custom-tailored, timely responses and information.

Additionally, within this complex academic medical center hierarchy, it is generally insufficient for the new leader to rely solely on having their immediate supervisor's trust and respect. Getting things done will also depend on them earning the trust and respect of other senior leaders, many of which they likely do not report to directly. As an example, a new department chair in a college of medicine is likely directly supervised by the Dean of the College of Medicine. But if the department has a residency program and conducts research, the chair may also be accountable to the Director of Graduate Medical Education and the Vice Chancellor for Research. Similarly, the chair will likely have accountability to a Vice President for Clinical Administration.

To successfully develop and navigate relationships with a variety of senior leaders, and to follow well in the most effective way, we believe new leaders would benefit from attending to the preferences and tendencies of their supervisor(s). We make the distinction between preferences and tendencies because preferences are typically more explicit. Often someone will express their preferences, whereas tendencies may be unconscious behaviors that require deductive inferences. Let's unpack this a bit.

As an example, imagine a new leader's preferred approach to problem solving is to engage in a lot of brainstorming. As such, the new leader may assume that in bringing a problem to their supervisor, the supervisor will be willing to collaboratively discuss a range of possible solutions and strategies, and then provide guidance on reaching the best strategy. However, suppose the supervisor prefers and anticipates their reports always come prepared with alternative solutions?

Due to their style differences, the new leader may perceive the supervisor to be disinterested, stifling creativity. Keep in mind, too, that the supervisor may be perceiving the new leader as unable to derive their own solutions! The supervisor may say at the conclusion of such a discussion, "the next time we meet to discuss a problem, please have two or three possible solutions to present." The savvy new leader should recognize this direction as the supervisor's preferred way of working, and then meet the supervisor's expectation moving forward.

But what happens when the supervisor doesn't express their preference? Say for example the supervisor turns away during the conversation, seems fidgety, or even gives a terse reply to the new leader. That's where the new leader's observation abilities need to come in - to analyze their supervisor's behavior and *infer* their preferences. Doing this requires the new leader to be deliberate about behavioral observations, and astute in their deductive reasoning. Inference is essentially

---

[1] Made popular from the 1996 movie, Jerry Maguire. Crowe, C. (Director). (1996). *Jerry Maguire* [Film]. TriStar Pictures.

developing hypotheses to explain what has been observed (e.g., explanations for why a behavior was exhibited). These skills are used widely across the academic medical center in teaching, clinical care, and research, and as such should likely be familiar to the new leader. We encourage the new leader to apply these skills in analyzing their supervisor(s)' interactions, behaviors, and tendencies.

Let's return to our example of the new leader and their supervisor who have different problem-solving styles. The new leader could easily infer from the observable behaviors that their supervisor is disinterested or upset. This is a key moment for the new leader. Rather than becoming reactive or judgmental, the new leader would do well instead to approach the situation with curiosity. The new leader could ask a question to substantiate their inference, such as, "For future meetings, how would you like to discuss problems that I am grappling with?" A question such as this invites an open dialogue with the supervisor, producing clear expectations for future conversations. As the old saying goes, "be curious, not furious."

It can be natural to shy away from this process for fear of making a wrong inference or drawing a wrong conclusion. This is a legitimate concern. If the new leader misses the mark, they can try a different approach at the next meeting and re-evaluate their supervisor's responses. Another approach is to ask others who report to this supervisor what communication and engagement strategies they have found useful. Gather data, try things out, see what gets traction, and keep going from there.

Lastly, it is important to clarify that being a good follower does not mean being spineless, blindly following, or sacrificing one's own integrity. Our point is that if the new leader wants to accomplish things beyond their span of positional control, they will need to build trust and credibility in all directions of the organization's hierarchy. A key to this includes the willingness to set one's own agenda, approach, or ego aside and follow others at certain times. Based on your role, in most situations you will lead, guide, direct, and inspire. But there will be times where the new leader's willingness to follow will in fact strengthen their ability to lead.

Courageous Followership

Blindly following, as noted above, squelches credibility. The new leader who does this with frequency becomes known as a "yes" person, willing to follow without asking questions, challenging anything or anyone, and leading their own unit without any thoughtfulness. They may be viewed as "agreeable" but entirely unhelpful.

To combat this outcome, a good follower must have the mettle to engage in crucial conversations, provide tough feedback, retain moral courage, or to speak frankly to senior leadership. Ira Chaleff addresses these and numerous other followership issues in his book, "The Courageous Follower." As he states:

> Courage is a prerequisite to healthy relationships and a fulfilling life. Courageous leaders and followers working together sow seeds. When circumstances do not let them reap the harvest themselves, they leave the soil enriched by their integrity and commitment for the next planting. [1, p. 236]

A good follower pushes back appropriately, sets healthy boundaries, points out dysfunctions, navigates harmful organizational processes and behaviors, and has the courage to say what needs to be said. Equally, a good leader has the courage to receive feedback from a courageous follower, to be open to new ideas and changes, and to not take resistance personally. As a new leader, we encourage you to be both.

Leading Up

In addition to courageously following, the new leader also has a job to do. And part of the skill of effective leadership is knowing how to achieve goals by engaging the support of those above in the hierarchy. In other words, appropriately influencing others with more positional power and authority to get things done. This is often referred to as "leading up," and it's an inherently important followership skill for the emerging leader wanting to function successfully in academic medical center environment.

While the emerging leader may not possess total positional control, they do possess a number of forms of influence. As we noted above, helping their supervisor(s) succeed is one form of influence, as being a high performer often yields the benefits of reward for the supervisor, oneself, and one's unit. Consider, too, the following influence strategies famously identified by Robert Cialdini [2], that the new leader (or anyone) may have at their disposal:

- Reciprocity—Influence acquired through a quid pro quo agreement. "I'll scratch your back and you scratch mine."
- Commitment/Consistency—In the workplace, people typically want to be reliable. Influence can be acquired by working with this tendency in others and securing agreements.
- Social Proof—Influence attained through power in numbers. For example, "Lots of our competitors are providing [x] with great success, so we should consider doing it as well."
- Authority—Similar to legitimate (positional) power, authority is influence based on being an "authority figure" because of one's title, social stature, and even professional clothing, etc. For example, drivers are much more apt to pay attention to a uniformed police officer directing traffic than a civilian in street clothes trying to do the same.
- Liking—Influence that is developed through relationship building and rapport. This can work directly or even indirectly. Film actor Tom Hanks can influence people he never meets, as he is commonly viewed to be a "really nice guy."
- Scarcity—Influence that is generated by the risk or potential risk of lack. When COVID-19 first reached the United States, the perceived risk of a toilet paper shortage created an actual shortage as people horded supplies.

The punchline here is that the new leader can navigate various situations with lots of options. For example, consider a department chair who is actively engaged in supporting the Chief Medical Officer (CMO), even though they have no reporting relationship. The CMO has numerous challenging relationships they need to manage. However, the chair's expertise, commitment, and rapport they provide makes the CMO's life easier. Because of their helpfulness and collaborative style, the chair has some influence with the CMO.

As another example, consider an IT director who influences the Chief Information Officer to purchase certain software for the hospital. The IT director points out that 14 of their 15 peer institutions are using the software with great ROI (social proof), and the software company is offering a 15% discount on purchases within the next 8 weeks (scarcity). Cialdini's influence strategies offer a myriad of combinations in which to be both a helpful, impactful follower and an effective leader.

A Note on Manipulation

It could be easy to look at these forms of influence and see how they might be used for self-serving purposes rather than for the greater good. And they could be. We have, unfortunately, in our careers seen people deploy such strategies, manipulating others for personal gain.

However, we have also seen that, in most cases, the manipulator will reap what they sow. No one likes to be played, and in the pressure filled, life or death environment of an academic medical center, there is very little patience for such gamesmanship. We encourage the new leader to consider utilizing these tools while treading lightly. Strategic and political rapport building to help one's unit be successful while also promoting the greater good of the institution is far different from choreographed, cunning maneuvers for one's own self-gain.

Following your Followers: Servant Leadership

Another aspect of being a good follower is the new leader's willingness to *follow those they lead*. This may seem like an odd idea, but for the roots of this concept we turn to Robert K. Greenleaf, who in 1964 founded what has become known as the Greenleaf Center for Servant Leadership.

During his career in corporate America, Greenleaf recognized that the command-and-control style of leadership, popularized through the industrial age, was becoming outdated and less helpful. The workplace was evolving into the information age, and the workforce was changing and becoming much more diverse and knowledge-based.

Greenleaf's research culminated with the development of the Servant Leadership model. As he states, "The servant-leader is servant first... It begins with the natural feeling that one wants to serve, to serve first" Greenleaf [3]. When a leader supports, develops, and champions their people *first*, the outcomes will be greater, as will the commitment of the followers. Being willing to follow those you lead signals you are open to sharing power and decision-making, that you value the contributions of all, and that you invite and support a culture of collaboration.

Another way to think about servant leadership is for the new leader to consider and treat their followers as their most important resource. To illustrate, imagine developing a relationship with a wealthy benefactor. The unit's development officer believes the benefactor is prepared to make a donation to the new leader's unit in the tens of millions of dollars. How the new leader thinks about and engages with that donor is likely different than how they might interact with a colleague they bump into in the hallway. This may sound pedantic, yet we as humans consciously or unconsciously choose to engage with different people in different ways. But, as a former coaching client of co-author, Rob, once stated, "I treat my team as if they are my most important customers." She went on to clarify that by engaging her team with the utmost respect and highest priority, they perform at their highest, making her life far easier and the success of the division that much better.

The key to being a servant leader is to effectively lead through an active, engaged, support focused, and service-oriented mindset.[2] The Servant Leadership model states that if the leader supports someone to be their very best, it will benefit not only the person, but also the team, the unit, and the entire organization.

Along these lines, a very important skill that we see effective leaders exhibit is that of giving credit to others. This can sometimes be hard to do, especially in the hierarchy of the academic medical center where one's success may determine future opportunities and positions. However, effective academic medical center leaders understand that no one achieves success on their own and that all parties involved deserve recognition.

To some this may seem like common sense, to others perhaps trivial. But everyone appreciates approval and recognition. Whether acknowledging the contributions of one's supervisor, the success of an initiative, or the individual contributors who elevate the unit's performance; being deliberate, sincere, and consistent with the public and private distribution of credit is one of the most important and effective skills a leader can adopt. We encourage every leader to spread acknowledgement and praise both widely and routinely.

Following Good Leaders

An effective strategy for getting better at leadership is to emulate what you see effective leaders do. And an excellent source for inspiration is the many current leaders in one's academic medical center. This sounds simple, but since no two people will manifest an attribute or skill the exact same way, we recommend the new leader not just copy, but adopt and adapt what they see effective leaders do to fit their own style. As a new leader, we encourage you to employ the deliberate observation skills we noted previously, watching how effective leaders act and the responses they generate from followers (positive and negative), including your own.

---

[2] These are all, by the way, actions the new leader has control over. Being a servant leader does not mean giving up power, influence, or authority.

To determine the attributes and behaviors to emulate, engage in a reverse engineering process. For example, consider a leader that you perceive to be a "really good listener." You might note that when you speak with them, they appear attentive, they make you feel important or valued, or they give you the sense they truly care about you. These descriptors are perceptions. The trick is to identify what actual *behaviors* the leader exhibits that generate your perceptions (e.g., lots of eye contact, pausing, inviting gestures or body position, affirming nods, clarifying back to you what they heard, empathizing, etc.). It is these *behaviors* that sparked the thinking, feelings, or actions in yourself and others, and as a result, the ones you might consider incorporating into your own leadership repertoire.

Historical leaders are another great source to explore for leadership lessons. We both enjoy reading biographies and historical non-fiction about leaders. As a new leader you may have a favorite historical leader, or you may read about several and develop a composite set of skills to inform your leadership approach. Often people look to historical leaders who have achieved prominence on the world stage, but they could just as easily be local, well regarded community leaders. We encourage new leaders to consider both as part of their research.

Irrespective of the size and scope of a leader's historical impact, we have gleaned a few common generalities from our reading and application. In our experience, great leaders typically:

- are purposeful, in fact they possess almost a singular resolve that is well-beyond themselves or their self-interests.
- are audacious in their vision and pursue it relentlessly.
- inspire others to "take up the vision" as well.
- exhibit amazing skills of communication, often as great orators, writers, or creators.
- take a long view of events, history, and their role in it.
- are resilient in the face of adversity, uncertainty, and ambiguity, and don't let failure deter their pursuit of an ultimate purpose or vision.

Ask any successful, long tenured leader why they lead the way they do, and they will likely tell you the story of the leader or leaders they learned from. As an emerging leader, understand that one of your greatest resources for learning to lead are other successful leaders. We encourage you to discover these leaders, living or historical, tested and refined in the trenches of leadership, and follow their lead.

Concluding Thoughts

As we close this chapter, we return to our opening premise that learning to follow is foundational to good leadership. We've discussed how an emerging leader can be an effective follower of those above them in the hierarchy, while still achieving their leadership responsibilities and goals at the unit level. We examined the role that leaders have in following (serving) those they lead, achieving success by helping others be successful. Lastly, we offered that one of the best ways to learn to lead well is by following the approaches of other successful leaders. There are innumerable good leaders working in academic medical centers, in other sectors, and throughout history to inspire your leadership journey. Our hope for you is that one day, other emerging leaders will look to you for the same inspiration.

How Do I Get Started?

It may seem counterintuitive to think that good leading involves following. Hollywood continues to depict the leader as the hero, overcoming unimaginable barriers to achieve success and save the day for others. Back on earth, good leadership is more about showing you care, listening with curiosity, and being open to following others' ideas and direction. You can start being a good leader by first figuring out how to be a good follower.

Coaching questions to ask yourself:
- Am I willing to do what it takes to lead in a complex environment (be a good follower, work with politics, identify and leverage key influencers, etc.)?
- What am I *not* willing to do in terms of being a follower?
- What surprised me most about what I read in this chapter? How does that inform what I might work on first?
- When does my ego get in the way of my or my team's success?
- What concerns me most about being a leader who follows? Why?
- What stories have I told myself about what it means to be a good leader, and what parts might I now adjust?
- Do I have a couple of leaders in mind (living or historical) that I can start to study?
- Are there one or two current leaders at my academic medical center that I could ask to mentor me in my leadership role? Why would I select them, and what would I like to learn from them?

Curious to learn more?
1. Caleb Leung, Amanda Lucas, Peter Brindley, Shellie Anderson, Jason Park, Ashley Vergis, Lawrence M. Gillman, Followership: A review of the literature in healthcare and beyond, *Journal of Critical Care*, Volume 46, 2018, Pages 99–104, ISSN 0883–9441, https://doi.org/10.1016/j.jcrc.2018.05.001.
2. Chaleff, I. (2009). The courageous follower: Standing up to & for our leaders (third ed.). Berrett-Koehler.
3. Greenleaf, R. K. (2015). The Servant as Leader. The Greenleaf Center for Servant Leadership; rev Edition.
4. Kramer, R., & Mauro, M. (2020). Leading Up. In Management and Leadership Skills for Medical Faculty and Healthcare Executives (pp. 183–190). Springer.
5. Riggio, R. E., Chaleff, I., & Lipman-Blumen, J. (Eds.). (2008). The Art of Followership: How Great Followers Create Great Leaders and Organizations. Jossey-Bass.
6. Titus, S., & Sanaghan, P. (2021, August 5). The Case for Good Followership on Campuses. Inside Higher Ed; Inside Higher Ed. https://www.insidehighered.com/advice/2021/08/05/importance-not-only-good-leaders-also-good-followers-opinion
7. Whitlock, J. (2013). The value of active followership. *Nursing management*, 20(2).

References

1. Chaleff I. The courageous follower: standing up to & for our leaders. 3rd ed. Berrett-Koehler; 2009.
2. Cialdini RB. Influence, new and expanded: the psychology of persuasion. Harper Business; 2021.
3. Greenleaf RK. The servant as leader. The Greenleaf Center for Servant Leadership; rev Edition; 2015.

Understanding (and Following) the Academic Medical Center's "Chain of Command"

12

The founding director of the physical therapy education program that co-author, Kyle, attended was a retired major in the U.S. military. The students who attended the program during her 10 years as director knew of her oft-repeated directive to "follow the chain of command." This command became so seared in Kyle's brain that over 40 years later he can still unequivocally say that it is the only thing he remembers from his formative professional education. Moreover, it has proven time and time again to be the one of the best pieces of advice he ever received!

The guidance seems so simple on the surface, but the wisdom contained therein has proven to be profound. Regardless, we are continuously amazed at how many people either don't know about this advice or know of it and still chose not to follow it. In this chapter we will explore the benefits of recognizing and utilizing this important cultural norm.

Chain of Command

Let's begin by being clear about the definition of "chain of command" [1, 2]. The concept is most often associated with organizations that exhibit a hierarchical organizational structure. This construct can sometimes get a bad rap as it is associated with "top down" leadership. We are not attempting to weigh its merits, only to acknowledge that, like any organizational model, a hierarchical model has its pros and cons [3]. The chain of command is simply a representation of an organization's authority hierarchy, generally depicted in an organizational chart. The resultant supervisory responsibilities and relationships in the chart are often referred to as the "reporting structure."

While usually not evident in the organizational chart, chain of command also implies the scope or span of each position's decision-making authority. Leadership and managerial positions are often defined by levels, being the "top" (e.g., President, Provost, Senior Executives/Vice Presidents, Chief Medical Officers, Deans), the "middle" (e.g., Associate Deans, Associate Provosts, Chairs, Department Heads), and "front/first line" (e.g., Medical Directors, Nurse Managers, Administrative Supervisors, Division Chiefs). In essence, the chain of command should provide clarity of role levels and locations in the organization, as well as the relationship of any given role to the others in the system. It is important to understand, as well, that when we use the term "chain of command" as it pertains to the academic medical center, we do so not solely to depict direct supervisory relationships, but as importantly to identify who needs to be informed about a given decision or outcome.

Successfully Navigating the Chain of Command in Your Academic Medical Center

We noted in the last chapter that because of loosely coupled, matrixed units, "every boss has a boss" (maybe more than one), and have accountability to other leaders, even if not in the direct chain of command. So, while it may seem obvious that leaders would understand and follow the chain of command, the organizational structure of the academic medical center can present nuances that can make clarity difficult for novice leaders.

New leaders who find themselves having "violated" the chain of command have typically done so due to inexperience or ignorance navigating the academic medical center's convolution of characteristics and nuances. For example, the new leader may not fully consider how a decision in their unit will impact another team, and therefore may not think to inform or engage the leader of another unit. Sometimes a new leader doesn't realize a decision they make is important enough (or they simply forget) to communicate it to their supervisor. In these cases, the new leader does not yet fully understand the organization's hierarchical context, and therefore (inadvertently) does not follow the chain of command. It usually takes only one episode to illuminate the value, importance, and impact of following the structure.

Make no mistake, the academic medical center is *highly* hierarchical. Deliberately choosing not to follow the chain of command, especially if done repeatedly, is an egregious offense, and one that senior leadership will tire of quickly. Implementing key decisions without counsel, failing to inform senior leadership of pending outcomes (especially public and/or negative ones), or disregarding their supervisor's guidance can lead to calamitous outcomes for the new leader, their unit, and potentially the organization.

To effectively navigate the chain of command, we recommend following a few simple steps. These recommendations might also be considered to help you become more politically savvy. In either case, recognize which choices you make yield successful outcomes, and which could become career derailers.

The first step is to always give your supervisor a "heads up" about a decision, situation, or outcome that may eventually come their way. Keep in mind that in large organizations like academic medical centers, it is not unusual to have multiple individuals "above you" in the hierarchy that may need to know such information. However, do not assume that you should be the one informing everyone in the chain.

It's best for you to inform your immediate supervisor and clarify whether they will inform others in the chain, or if they would prefer for you to do so.

Use good discretion, but it is typically better to inform people than not to do so. No one likes surprises. As an example, an academic medical center dean recalls a situation when a vice-chancellor (who was both a supervisor and friend) called to ask her if she knew that someone in her college was a finalist candidate for a leadership position at another institution. She did not, and when she raised this with the faculty member in question, the response was he had not thought it was important to communicate about his candidacy unless and until he was offered the job. The dean felt embarrassed to not know about this situation, even though other senior leaders knew. She found herself questioning what her supervisor thought of her leadership, as well as wondering what else the faculty member may not be telling her.

The second step is, no matter how convenient or efficient it might be to skip a level in the chain of command, do not. What you potentially gain in expediency, you will lose in long-term trust. As an illustration, a college dean experienced one of his direct reports (a program director) going to the dean of another college to inquire about having their program join his college. When the "home" dean confronted their program director with this information, the program director indicated that they were "just trying to gather information" so they could speak with him later about the topic. The dean interpreted this as a veiled excuse, and the experience significantly damaged the trust between the two parties.

Despite your best efforts, a time will likely come when you will find yourself having failed to inform someone of something important or having otherwise gotten yourself in over your head. It's important to remember that in a complex bureaucratic organization like an academic medical center, this is bound to happen. It's equally important to fix the problem immediately. Take ownership, apologize if necessary, and get the correct person(s) in the loop. A bad beginning does not have to have a bad ending.

Who's in This Chain, Anyway?

So-called "violations" of the chain of command also play out in less obvious manners than the situations described above. For example, consider the leader who is recognized as accomplished and approachable. She routinely has individuals seeking her out for advice. She may even have individuals from other units coming to her. It can be flattering to be approached for advice. However, be mindful to the organizational hierarchy and consider the politics involved.

To illustrate, imagine you are approached by an individual wanting validation that their rocky relationship with their supervisor is due to the supervisor's (your colleague's) poor leadership. Tread very lightly. Taking responsibility to solve someone else's problem when it is not within your formal position or authority to do so can put you in an awkward position. You might listen, help the individual "reframe" the situation, or brainstorm strategies on how to broach the topic with their supervisor. In any case, be cautious not to give assent to an individual's perceptions, or to say anything that could be interpreted as disparaging of the other supervisor. Despite the temptation to help solve their problem or validate their feelings, the goal is, instead, to encourage the individual to make their own decision, such as returning to their supervisor for a candid conversation.

In this regard, consider a concept put forward by Steven Sample in his book, *The Contrarian's Guide to Leadership* [4]. In his role of University President, Sample valued and invited open communication, particularly between himself and the members of the university community. This strategy allowed him to learn a great deal about members of the organization, to get clear on work that needed to be done, while at the same time conveying a sense of approachability and accessibility.

Sample described his approach as "open communication with structured decision making" [5], noting he was cautious not to let this style put him at cross-purposes with the other members of his leadership team. Hence, his insistence on "structured decision making," so as not to let accessibility be misconstrued as pre-empting others' decision-making authority. He notes,

> Under this rubric, everyone in the organization is free to communicate directly with everyone else in the organization, with the explicit caveat that *any and all commitments, allocations, and decisions will be made strictly through the hierarchy* (italics in the original) [5].

As Sample implies, there is nothing inherently wrong with talking to the president, or any other person in the academic medical center. We encourage you, however, to inform your supervisor of your desire to have these conversations, to obtain their prior approval, and when possible, to also share the outcomes of the conversation. Similarly, as a leader in the organization, be mindful to direct those who seek you out to the appropriate decision-making authority, as warranted, before approaching you.

Another aspect to consider involves formal communication. Specifically, "who needs to know what?" and perhaps even more importantly, "when do they need to know it?" As examples, imagine you just finalized plans with a major donor to renovate a research lab, or just hired a well-known physician to assume the role of division chief. In the interest of efficiency, it may be tempting to inform everyone in the chain (or even the organization) at once. However, prior to an announcement becoming public, it is important to alert, first, those who have ultimate authority over the unit (e.g., Dean, Chancellor) and second, those who may be contacted about the announcement (for example, by the media). Furthermore, inquire if the Chancellor, hospital CEO, or members of the Board of Trustees should be informed in advance about an important announcement.

Identify who, by individual or group, is in the chain of communication and tailor both your message and the timing of the message accordingly to their unique needs. Updates to different populations may roll out over a few hours, or it could occur over days or weeks. In the academic medical center, major announcements are typically managed by the public relations or strategic communications department, but smaller announcements may be handled by your own team. In either case, we encourage you to be an active participant in the process.

Lastly, new leaders need to remember that they act as a conduit of information. Their flow of communication needs to go both up to their supervisor(s), and down to the members of their unit. Just as the Board of Trustees does not appreciate hearing an announcement at the same time as the public, members of your unit, who are often those directly affected by the news, do not appreciate it either.

The Art of Advocating

Advocating for oneself, for someone else, for their unit, or for a strategic decision is a common component of the leader's job. The new leader needs to be cognizant of the chain of command when engaging in advocacy. However, advocating may be more nuanced depending on the topic and specific variables.

Take for example a division chief who would like to help advance the work of a rising star researcher in their unit. Their college has a new Associate Dean for Research (ADR), and the division chief is concerned that because of the ADR's limited tenure, they may not have an established relationship with the university's Vice Chancellor for Research. The division chief might be tempted to go around the ADR for efficiency's sake. However, by starting with the ADR, that person can in turn pull in the Dean, and together they can create a unified front, advocating with much greater effectiveness to the Vice Chancellor.

What appears at first to be the efficient choice may actually be slower and yield weaker results in the end. The ADR and the Dean may not be happy with the division chief's action of going rogue, access to the Vice Chancellor may be denied, and (regardless of the outcome) trust is damaged. The advice here is to know your role, respect the position of others in the hierarchy, and take politically astute actions.

Similarly, if a dean wanted to advocate for one of their faculty members to receive a courtesy appointment in another college, they could contact the department chair in the other college directly. However, this action might be viewed as using their position authority to "strong arm" the department chair. It would be more effective and appropriate for the dean to first contact the dean of the other college to ask if that dean would either speak with their department chair or connect them with the inquiring dean.

Other Chains of Communication at the Academic Medical Center

Many activities within the academic medical center are governed by various regulations and laws that define communication rules, requirements, and reporting structures. We bring this to your attention to clearly distinguish reporting "requirements" from "voluntary" adherence associated with the chain of command. If you are not familiar with these regulations from your previous clinical or teaching activities, we urge you to seek further information on the following, as they will likely become relevant at some point in your leadership tenure:

- Health Insurance Portability and Accountability Act (HIPAA)[1]
- Family Educational Rights and Privacy Act (FERPA)[2]
- Ethical access to clinical research data[3]
- Mandatory reporting laws[4]

There's one other important consideration about the chain of command, as it pertains to the primary mission of healthcare delivery. There are far too many real examples of patient care gone awry, regrettably, sometimes with significant consequences, due to "chain of command" norms limiting people to feel safe speaking up if they see something wrong. Many academic medical centers have created systems and procedures whereby *every* employee, regardless of job title, is empowered to file patient safety alerts for any imminent or potential risk situation. [6] Others have implemented a training program called Team Strategies and Tools to Enhance Performance and Patient Safety (TeamSTEPPS®), [7, 8] developed by the Agency for Healthcare Research and Quality (AHRQ) in collaboration with the U.S. Department of Defense. The training provides evidenced-based information and strategies to improve communication and teamwork skills to reduce medical errors and improve patient safety.

The point is that every member of the healthcare team, of the entire academic medical center for that matter, is responsible for patient safety. In this regard, there should not be a chain of command, but rather a team of people unified and inextricably linked to secure every patient's safety.

The "Secret of Life"

We opened by telling you about Kyle's early professional experience with his program director. He often jokes that this person was so insistent on giving and repeating the advice, "follow the chain of command," that he came to understand this as not just a directive, but the very "secret of life." While obviously a humorous exaggeration, you'd be amazed at how many problems can be avoided, and how many relationships strengthened, by adhering to this simple tenet. Your leadership journey will be far more successful if you do so, as well.

---

[1] Centers for Disease Control and Prevention. Public Health Professionals Gateway. Health Insurance Portability and Accountability Act of 1996 (HIPAA) Available at https://www.cdc.gov/phlp/publications/topic/hipaa.html.

[2] U.S. Department of Education. Family Educational Rights and Privacy Act (FERPA). Available at https://www2.ed.gov/policy/gen/guid/fpco/ferpa/index.html.

[3] Choi HJ, Lee MJ, Choi CM, et al. Establishing the role of honest broker: bridging the gap between protecting personal health data and clinical research efficiency. *PeerJ*. 2015;3:e1506. Published 2015 Dec 17. doi:10.7717/peerj.1506. Available at https://www.ncbi.nlm.nih.gov/pmc/articles/PMC4690386/.

[4] Thomas R, Reeves M. Mandatory Reporting Laws. [Updated 2021 Jul 15]. In: StatPearls [Internet]. Treasure Island (FL): StatPearls Publishing; 2022 Jan-. Available at https://www.ncbi.nlm.nih.gov/books/NBK560690/.

How Do I Get Started?

For some new leaders, it can be tough to go from working with great auton-omy to now keeping in close communication with their supervisor(s), direct reports, and others. The work of communicating is just that, work. Expect this new reality and recognize that the needs and demands of being in a formal leadership role require you to be more aware of the implications and conse-quences of communication. Ensure effective and consistent communication up and down the chain of command.

Coaching questions to ask yourself:
- Who do I need to keep abreast of my and my team's work? How do they want to be updated, and how frequently?
- What types of issues should be elevated to my reporting chain? What types of issues should I share with my team?
- Are there certain topics I should not be sharing "up" and/or "down?"
- Before I take action outside of my typical chain of command, what factors do I need to consider?
- Who do I know that understands the political environment of my unit and reporting chain, and can provide me insights before I make decisions?

Curious to learn more?
1. Ayers, A. A. (n.d.). Follow the Chain of Command. The Journal of Urgent Care Medicine; JUCM. Retrieved February 20, 2022, from https://www.jucm.com/follow-chain-command/
2. Chaleff, I. (2009). The Courageous Follower: Standing Up to and for Our Leaders. Berrett-Koehler Publishers.
3. Hesselbein, F. (2013). Hesselbein On Leadership. Jossey-Bass.
4. Kaplan, G. S. November 9, 2018. Building a Culture of Transparency in Health Care. Harvard Business Review; Harvard Business Review. https://hbr.org/2018/11/building-a-culture-of-transparency-in-health-care
5. Stevens T. (2020) Political Savvy. In: Viera A., Kramer R. (eds) Manage-ment and Leadership Skills for Medical Faculty and Healthcare Execu-tives. Springer, Cham. https://doi.org/10.1007/978-3-030-45425-8_21
6. Strategies for Effective Communication in Health Care. (2021, September 29). Tulane University School of Public Health and Tropical Medicine; Tulane University School of Public Health and Tropical Medicine. https://publichealth.tulane.edu/blog/communication-in-healthcare/

References

1. Chain of Command. The Strategic CFO Blog. Available at https://strategiccfo.com/chain-of-command/, https://www.indeed.com/career-advice/career-development/chain-of-command
2. Indeed Editorial Team. February 22, 2021. What is a chain of command? (definition and explanation). *Indeed Career Guide Blog*. Available at https://www.indeed.com/career-advice/career-development/chain-of-command
3. Understanding Organizational Structures. SHRM. Available at https://www.shrm.org/resourcesandtools/tools-and-samples/toolkits/pages/understandingorganizationalstructures.aspx
4. Sample SB. The Contrarian's guide to leadership. San Francisco, CA: Jossey-Bass; 2002.
5. Sample SB. The Contrarian's guide to leadership (p. 32). San Francisco, CA: Jossey-Bass; 2002.
6. Kaplan GS. Building a culture of transparency in healthcare. Harvard business review. Harv Bus Rev. 2018, November 9; https://hbr.org/2018/11/building-a-culture-of-transparency-in-health-care
7. Agency for Healthcare Research and Quality. TeamSTEPPS. Available at https://www.ahrq.gov/teamstepps/index.html
8. King HB, Battles J, Baker DP, et al. TeamSTEPPS™: Team Strategies and Tools to Enhance Performance and Patient Safety. In: Henriksen K, Battles JB, Keyes MA, et al., editors. Advances in patient safety: new directions and alternative approaches, Performance and Tools, vol. 3. Rockville, MD: Agency for Healthcare Research and Quality (US); 2008. Available at https://www.ncbi.nlm.nih.gov/books/NBK43686/.

The Value of "Invisible" Leadership 13

When people think of a "leader" they most often think of the current, oft-quoted public ambassador of the unit or organization. This is one aspect of the leader's role. As the "face" of the organization, the leader's public presence, whether inward (to the members of the academic medical center) or outward (to the public, donors, alumni, community), sends a strong message about the "health and wellness" of the organization and its value to the academic medical center and community.

Though this aspect of a leader's performance is what is visible to others, much of the leader's work is unseen or confidential. This is not to imply that leadership should involve secrecy. Rather, an inherent aspect of leadership is often having first-hand access to information (which at the time may not be for others' consumption), as well as at times dealing with information that should always remain confidential.

Behind the Scenes Is Often the "Scene"

Emerging leaders may be surprised how much of the role this aspect comprises. What happens behind the scenes, in our estimation, easily constitutes 40–50% of the leader's work. We bring this to your attention because it is quite feasible that if you are an effective leader, many members of the academic medical center won't know (and shouldn't know) the significant contributions you make.

The majority of this behind-the-scenes work involves three things: money (budget), people (personnel management), and change (transformation/innovation). The driver, and critical skill, for accomplishing much of the work is brokering, or negotiating with others. Let's unpack these categories a little more.

K. P. Meyer, R. Kramer, *Taking the Lead*,
https://doi.org/10.1007/978-3-031-16711-9_13

Money

The leader may be the only, or one of only a few members of the unit involved with other senior organizational officials in the early stages of budget planning. We have touted the value of the leader demonstrating transparency in their interactions. And ultimately, the outcome of budget planning and decisions should be transparent. But if the actual planning process was conducted with *all* members of the organization from the outset, it would likely create unnecessary confusion and anxiety rather than improve the process.

Consider, for example, your public academic medical center being confronted with a 10% budget reduction (not uncommon in this day and age). Reductions may be evenly distributed across all units, or they may be targeted to specific areas or initiatives. Often at the outset of the budget planning process, multiple scenarios are put forward for consideration and "stress testing." If a scenario emerges that calls for a larger percentage reduction for your unit, you might engage in an early series of negotiations to alter the plan or reduce its potential impact on your unit.

Concurrent with the initial campus level discussions, you would begin to consider how to make the reduction if it proved necessary to do so, investigating possible scenarios and the implications to your unit. You will almost certainly have conversations and deliberations with your supervisor(s), the person who manages the unit's finances, and perhaps other members of your executive team. However, engaging the broader membership of the unit too soon, particularly when a final decision has yet to be made, would likely not be interpreted as thoughtful planning, but more likely raise anxiety and create unnecessary discord.

Managing potential budget cuts is not the only example of confidential money issues you can expect to work on. Salary negotiations, determining annual salary distribution, investigating the financial implications of requests for space and personnel, and considerations regarding capital equipment and construction are but a few of the money related conversations that occur routinely. These conversations can extend over several months, if not longer. And at times, even when you think a final decision has been reached, it may be changed.

The leader's role in navigating and negotiating issues related to money is incredibly important to the success of the unit. *And* the leader needs to understand this work may never be fully understood or appreciated by the members of their unit.

People

Leaders expend a lot of behind-the-scenes time and energy on activities related to personnel management.[1] These activities literally span the full cycle from recruitment to termination. Much of the work may be thought of as handling "problems," and these do exist! Common examples include personal situations (i.e., medical

---

[1] "Personnel" typically refers to paid employees of the unit, but some leaders will also deal with similar issues pertaining to students, residents, or fellows.

conditions, family issues, home maintenance surprises, etc.), lapses in judgement, ethics, sexual misconduct, and issues of compliance or legality. This is by no means an exhaustive list but be aware you *can* expect people to present you with a myriad of concerns and issues.

Leading people, however, also comes with a lot of behind-the-scenes work dedicated to their growth and development. Examples include developmental coaching, mentoring, nominating high performers for awards, attending award ceremonies, securing funding for other's professional development, etc. Some of these actions may be public, but much of it happens behind closed doors. As Olympic and world champion Allyson Felix says, "Everyone sees the glory moments, but they don't see what happens behind the scenes" [1].

We have noticed that when new leaders first encounter personnel situations they often fall under the illusion that the goal is to solve the problem or give the needed direction as quickly as possible in order to get back to the "more important things" that need their attention. After many decades of doing this work, we have come to understand what now seems obvious: personnel issues (negative or positive) never go away, and they are not simply an occasional issue. Rather, regularly dealing with people *is* the real job of the leader—or at least a big part of it.

Also, as it pertains to personnel "problems," keep in mind that it is not solely your responsibility to fix them. In fact, it's not in your best interest to attempt to do so. The academic medical center is replete with individuals available to assist you. Depending on the nature of issue, you will possibly engage legal counsel, vice-chancellors, the chief compliance officer, the Title IX coordinator, the director of HR, the chief diversity officer, the chief financial officer, and a host of others.

It's far beyond the scope of this chapter to detail the interactions you will have with these individuals or offices, other than to reinforce the need for confidentiality with these advisors. We also want to emphasize that these experts are there to help you. Engage them *early* in the process, share complete information with them, and listen to their counsel. As the leader of your unit, it is certainly your prerogative to ask them questions, seek clarification, and have differing opinions, but we strongly caution you to not disregard their advice.

As we both have become more adept at helping many individuals negotiate favorable resolutions to some thorny personnel problems, we've come to appreciate that while difficult and at times exhausting, reaching a resolution (for both the individual and organization) can be one of the most rewarding aspects of leadership. And it happens primarily behind the scenes. We encourage you to value not only the public role and recognition, but perhaps even more, the experience of supporting and developing others to be successful. Even when it's not easily seen.

Change

We refer you to Chap. 16 for more detailed information about change management and your leadership role as a change agent. Here, we want to mention that change initiatives often begin with behind-the-scenes work. While we note that change initiatives should be transparent and evidenced-based, it is important to understand that transparency is most important when the initiative is ready for "prime time."

A change is generally preceded by a deliberative phase of behind-the-scenes planning, when the leader likely engages a small group of confidants, including the leader's executive or "Kitchen" cabinets, and other trusted mentors or supervisors. The goal of these conversations is refinement, to assist the leader in crystalizing their thinking and developing a plan that includes a strong case for the change. Elements include the rationale for the change, the process necessary to implement the change (including inviting and evaluating feedback), the strategy to introduce the proposed change (to the unit and/or the organization as necessary), and consideration of a pilot program, to gather additional evidence about the process for, and impact of, the proposed change. These deliberative conversations also provide the leader's inner circle with foreknowledge of the proposed change and the opportunity to support it.

While it's not a rule of thumb, we observe that leaders often have more ideas than they ever could (or should) implement. Consequently, during this deliberative phase, it is equally plausible that in bouncing their thoughts off a dependable group of advisors, the leader may decide to abandon what was initially considered to be a valuable idea. Brain-storming concepts in a safe environment such as this expands the leader's creativity and decision-making acumen.

You may be beginning to recognize that if the leader engages in this process with the entire unit on every possible idea, poor outcomes could emerge. A primary one being confusion or disarray, as the member's may be overwhelmed by a continuous "flood" of ideas. Some will take the leader's musings as directives, thus initiating what they think the leader desires, only to later have their efforts disregarded, shut down, or deemed unnecessary. In the name of transparency (or lack of self-regulation), the leader inadvertently undermines their own credibility. Additionally, when the leader provides wide-spread access into their early thinking and planning about a change, it can afford those who are more resistant to the change an extended period of time to develop strategies and coalitions to oppose it.

As a reminder, we are in favor of transparency pertaining to change initiatives, but only after generative and deliberative planning has occurred. Once the behind-the-scenes work yields a clear plan, including strategies for obtaining feedback and mitigating challenges, the leader can then openly and transparently reveal the strategy that has been developed up to this point.

Brokering

Brokering is akin to acting like an agent, connecting people with one another, talking with individuals about projects they might be interested in, and securing them career advancement opportunities. As leader, you will likely develop a broad understanding of the personnel, activities, and initiatives across campus, and often gain early access to information about new campus initiatives. A savvy leader will use this access to navigate and negotiate opportunities for those they lead. Put another way, brokering is using your boundary spanning skills (see Chap. 4) to connect the dots between your unit and the larger campus and university community.

Brokering also involves determining the content and veracity of negative feedback about members of your unit. Investigating these situations often reveals "two sides to the story." It is your responsibility to (1) address any unfounded complaints, and (2) when there is a legitimate issue, work collaboratively to develop strategies that address the consequences of unintended mistakes, ensuring appropriate improvement. In this regard, brokering involves protecting and developing those you lead.

As an example, early in co-author Kyle's career as a pediatric physical therapist, he received feedback from his mentor that a physician was irate about the poor quality of a patient examination Kyle had conducted. Rather than allow Kyle to be devastated by this early failure, his mentor (who was a seasoned developmental pediatrician) contacted the referring physician and assured him the outcome resulted from a misunderstanding about the referral, clarified that Kyle was an excellent physical therapist with great potential, and that Kyle would obtain the necessary information the physician was seeking. This brokering allowed Kyle to become acutely aware of the need to clarify expectations, and he never forgot the gesture on the part of his mentor. Over his subsequent years in administration, Kyle has gone on to intentionally provide similar outcomes for many others under his leadership.

The Art of Playing the Long Game

Another leadership responsibility that includes behind-the-scenes work is being the "strategic visionary" for the unit. In doing so, the leader will find themselves laying the groundwork for an aspirational future. Examples could include launching a new institute, developing a new degree program, securing funding for an endowed chair position, or engaging in a capital construction project. We call this "behind-the-scenes" work because the leader usually engages key individuals in what can often be the extensive process of getting a big initiative to the top of the organization's priorities list. This process tends to be non-linear, stopping and starting over months or years as situations and people change, and with the results usually not becoming "public" until the institution commits to move the initiative forward. As such, this critically important work requires considerable vigilance and perseverance.

We have found a few strategies that are effective for this type of foundation building work. Although we identify them as unique and sequential steps, they do inherently overlap. Please note, these suggestions can be useful for moving both your big ideas forward as well as for less substantial initiatives.

Step #1: Seed Your Idea

If you have an idea that you think is a good one, but you are not totally sure, vet the concept with a few trusted individuals (see the "deliberative phase" of change described earlier in the chapter). These could be trusted confidants, although we encourage you to also engage individuals with varied perspectives. At this point in the process, you don't need to be fully committed to the idea, but rather indicate you are contemplating it and would like their reactions.

Listen and watch carefully to their verbal and non-verbal feedback. Their responses will help you refine your idea by pointing out implications and consequences you had not previously considered, as well as help you gain a better understanding of components that may be supported. After refining your idea, then try sharing it with someone who has the ear of the supervisor (e.g., the key decision maker). Their feedback can help you gain further clarity whether or not your idea has the power to be supported and implemented.

Step #2: Speaking Your Plan into Existence

After seeding and refining your big idea with a small number of key stakeholders, you may observe the idea gaining traction. More people will be talking about it, and you can use this as a cue to share the idea with an increasingly wider range of constituents, including some who you anticipate may not be as favorable to your idea. If you meet opposition, you can point out that others have already offered their support.

In the academic medical center environment, ideas spread, especially good ideas. Look for opportunities at various meetings to indicate you are seriously considering the new initiative, and have garnered some early, favorable feedback. People will often respond that "they have heard about the idea through the grapevine." At which point you can also invite them to provide their thoughts and input. As momentum builds around good ideas (keep in mind, this may take many months or even years), people may lose sight of how the idea originated. A key moment is when someone else in the organization informs *you* about *your* original idea. Then you know it is getting closer to becoming a reality.

Step #3: Getting Your Idea on the "Agenda"

Political scientist John Kingdon provides useful insights on how things get on the federal policy agenda, using a metaphor of three-streams [2].

Kingdon identifies what he terms, the "problem stream," the "policy stream," and the "political stream." The problem stream is the issue that needs to be addressed/fixed by a policy (or for you, the new academic medical center leader, the big idea you need/want to get done). The policy stream contains myriad solutions from multiple groups of stakeholders. Kingdon notes that these solutions have often been around well before, and well after, the specific problem they attempt to address. As Kingdon notes, "more often, solutions search for problems" [3]. The political stream represents the will of the policy (decision) makers to address a given problem. Kingdon also notes that, "each of the streams has a life of its own, largely unrelated to the others" [4].

According to Kingdon, when these three streams flow together the item in question makes it to the agenda. That is, decision-makers decide (or are forced to decide) that *now* is the time to act because the problem has become paramount, and because readily available solutions exist.

As applied to your behind-the-scenes foundational work in the academic medical center, Kingdon's model is just as relevant. Present your vision (initiative) in a clear and compelling fashion, identifying not just the intended outcomes for your unit, but for the institution. Be adaptable, look for and be willing to engage partners. There may be others in the organization that have a similar problem or need, and they may have existing recommendations or solutions that would support your initiative.

The likelihood of getting your item on the institutional "agenda" will increase if you are willing to engage others in the planning, such that your outcome can also meet the needs of *other* units or important institutional goals. Lastly, work to make the decision "inevitable," by positioning everyone involved for success. One of the best strategies for getting things done in an academic medical center is to have your idea become an item on your supervisor's agenda.

Wait, What? A Note About "Getting Credit"

Before winding up this chapter, it is critical for your mental and emotional well-being to understand that people typically want not only to succeed, but to be recognized for their accomplishments. Herein lies the problem. You may spend much of your time doing important behind-the-scenes work and not necessarily be recognized for the outcomes. For example, your leadership managing a personnel issue may avert a potentially bad outcome or crisis. You can't tell anyone because of confidentiality and human resources considerations. And as is often true of prevention strategies, you can't take credit for what *didn't* happen.

Also, as it pertains to your role in introducing new ideas or initiatives, remember that perceptions shift the farther your proposed initiative moves on from the initial groundwork you laid. This is a common occurrence because (1) time diminishes memory, and (2) bringing big ideas to fruition is a team sport, so others will no doubt deserve recognition for the outcome as well. Behind-the-scenes work is exactly that. Locally, the activities you devote your time and energy to may be hard for members of your unit to see and fully appreciate. Thus, you may need to remind yourself periodically that the impact your leadership had on your unit and the institution may not be fully understood (or appreciated) until after you leave your position.

Periodically you will also need to remind yourself that the true meaning of success in leadership is not recognition, but accomplishment. You may not always get the credit you deserve in the moment, but don't let the need to get credit for a great idea or outcome get in the way of *actually achieving* the outcome. Do good work for good work's sake.

How Do I Get Started?

The idea of "leading from behind" can be a real challenge for some new leaders, while it may be natural and intuitive for others. A good first step is to take inventory of your new role. Find out what aspects of the role are public facing and what work is behind-the-scenes. We strongly encourage you not to guess on this, as it can have big, unwanted consequences. Talk to your supervisor, colleagues with experience in similar roles, mentors, and anyone else who may help you get as clear as possible on the role you have assumed. Key areas to explore include, but are not limited to:

- Competence: Given to requirements of this role, what skills or aptitudes do I need to develop?
- Decision-making: What topics should I involve others in, and which should I address on my own?
- Standards: What are the standards of excellence I have inherited for my unit, and what needs to be adjusted?
- Accountability: How do I hold my team accountable for their work, and how can they hold me accountable for mine?
- Clarifying Expectations: How well am I doing at clarifying expectations for all of the items, above? What can I do different/better?

This is not a simple process, but the further you can reveal the true needs of your new leadership role, the further you will be along the path to success.

Coaching questions to ask yourself:

- What problems or opportunities on my list do I see as high priority items that I may want to get on my supervisor's (or the institution's) radar?
- Who can I turn to for help and advice as I am getting started?
- If I don't yet have a Kitchen Cabinet, who would I like to be on it?
- How do I do my "background" work as leader and be sure my supervisor knows I am focusing on the right things in my role?
- Who have I seen that is good at these skills? What do they do well?
- How do I move an initiative forward and not make it about me?

Curious to learn more?

1. Fisher, R., Ury, W., & Patton, B. (2006). Getting to yes (2nd ed.). Penguin Putnam.
2. Galunic, C. (2020). Backstage leadership: The invisible work of highly effective leaders. Palgrave Macmillan.
3. Greenleaf, R. K. (2002). Servant leadership: A journey into the nature of legitimate power and greatness. Paulist Press.
4. Kingdon, J. W. (1984). Agendas, alternatives, and public policies. Boston: Little, Brown.
5. Rock, D. (2006). Quiet leadership: Help people think better—don't tell them what to do: six steps to transforming performance at work. New York: Collins.

References

1. Snowden S. November 18. Exclusive: Allyson Felix, the Best to Ever Do It. Ebony; Ebony; 2019. https://www.ebony.com/black-history/icons_legends/allyson-felix-olympics-interview/
2. Kingdon JW. Agendas, alternatives, and public policies. Louisville: Ron Newcomer & Associates; 1984.
3. Ibid, p. 91.
4. Ibid, p. 90.

The Leader's Role in Academic Medical Center Philanthropy

14

When we speak to new leaders about their role, seldom does fundraising rise to the top of the discussion. Even more so, when tasked with raising philanthropic support for their unit, the new leader's immediate response is generally similar and predictable, "I don't like asking people for money." While you may or may not be comfortable (or experienced) at this important skill, you will quickly learn that fundraising is an inherent part of your unit's success. It is important to understand both the process of fundraising and your potential role(s) within it. And, spoiler alert, your role has very little to do with asking for money.

The Basics of Philanthropy

By its very nature, the academic medical center is reliant on various forms of external funding support to accomplish its missions, and the impact of philanthropy on higher education is enormous. For example, over the next two decades it has been projected that baby boomers will collectively transfer over $30 trillion [1] in personal wealth to the next generation, and in fiscal year 2020 alone approximately $49.5 billion was given to higher education [2].

Because emerging leaders often have little interaction with philanthropists before assuming a leadership role, we thought it would be valuable to provide a short primer on the basics of philanthropy.

- The official names used for what you may have formerly called "fundraising" are "development" or "advancement."
- The development function in academic medical centers is often administered or managed by a dedicated person(s) from a Development or Advancement Office

K. P. Meyer, R. Kramer, *Taking the Lead*,
https://doi.org/10.1007/978-3-031-16711-9_14

or "Foundation" assigned to raise money for your academic unit. Your unit's "development officer(s)" serves as the liaison between your unit and this office.[1]

- The contract that establishes the relationship between the institution and the benefactor is called the "fund agreement" or "gift agreement." It establishes the amount and timeline for funding, as well as creates the conditions for its use.
- Philanthropic support generally falls into one of two types, *restricted* or *unrestricted* funds.
  - A restricted fund[2] has specifically outlined conditions for its use and can only be spent according to these conditions.
  - An unrestricted fund, sometimes called a "discretionary" fund, is much more flexible, and is intended to be used at the discretion of the individual(s) who have "spending authority" for the fund.
  - The benefactor will often establish the parameters for their support dependent on their specific goals. Consequently, most gifts are restricted funds.
- Philanthropic support can also be generally divided into one of two categories, *endowed* funds, and *expendable* funds.
  - An endowed fund invests the original principal, resulting in some portion of the interest being used annually to advance the purpose of the gift ("spendable net income"). Endowed funds are attractive to donors because they exist in perpetuity, and are generally "named," thus creating a legacy for the donor.
  - An expendable fund is more time-limited, and "spends down" the original gift based on the directives of the fund agreement (this may be over several years). Thus, when the money is gone, so too is the fund. Expendable funds are attractive to donors who may want to make a larger impact immediately.

The Leader's Role in Philanthropy

We don't want to oversimplify things, but from the new leader's perspective, we offer that working with philanthropists is actually pretty simple, if you understand the needs of your potential benefactors. Namely, they want to have a *clear* understanding of a *specific* problem, and typically prefer straightforward, direct solutions. They want to know how their funding will help achieve the solution, as well as any other outcomes that can be anticipated. Lastly, although it should probably go without saying, they want accurate information. It is in no one's interest to try to embellish a funding request, exaggerate the problem or over promise on the outcomes.

---

[1] Your unit may be charged an "advancement fee" (a flat fee, or a small percentage of a gift) to help fund the activities of the Development Office.

[2] A piece of advice: as the leader, if you can provide input to the donor about the fund agreement, asking them to consider the "broadest restrictions" to meet their goals will provide you the greatest latitude for future use. For example, if the donor wants to establish an endowed professorship pertaining to the education mission, a professorship (and fund agreement) that supports the advancement of teaching innovation and excellence, provides more "discretion" for the leader than a professorship that supports the advancement of teaching in molecular biology.

The result is that as the leader, you will typically do the explaining and your professional development officer will do the asking. Your role boils down to answering two basic questions for the donor:

1. What is the vision of my unit/project/cause? (Create a compelling story and future).
2. If you received a philanthropic investment, what would it enable you to do that you couldn't otherwise do with existing funding?

How well you answer these questions, more accurately, *how well you present the answers* to these questions, will to a large extent determine your success in securing philanthropic support. Your answers should be exciting, paint a vivid picture, and be forward thinking.

Preparing Your Proposal

A simple tool we have found useful in developing the answers to these questions is the "quad chart," [3] (see Fig. 14.1) which is often used to summarize research funding requests of federal agencies. It can also be readily adapted for proposals seeking philanthropic support. The basic elements of the chart include:

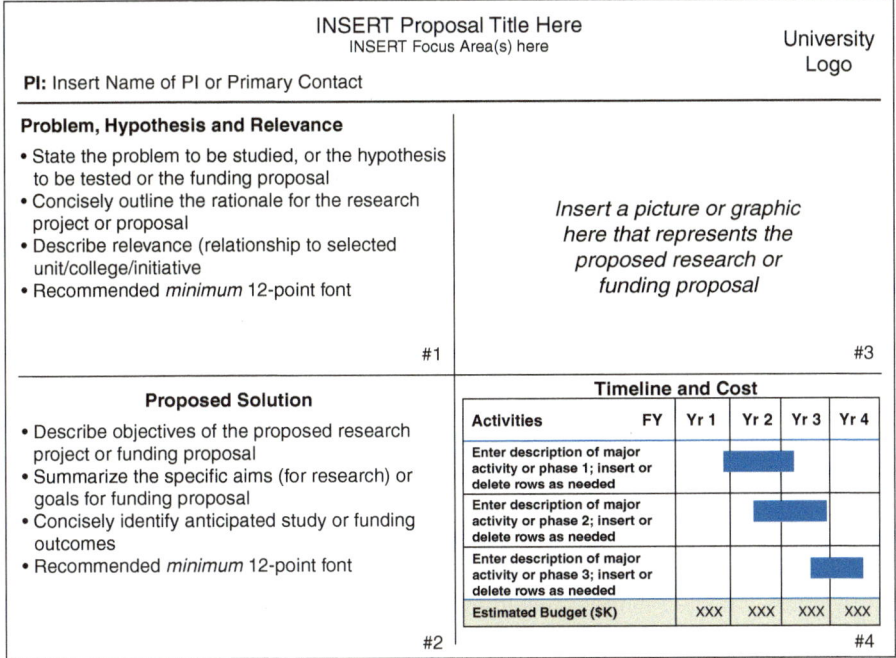

Fig. 14.1 Quad Chart Sample Template (The quads are numbered for explanatory purposes. You would not include the numbers in a final document)

- Quadrant 1: title, project description, summary statement defining the proposal and its relevance
- Quadrant 2: the proposal's benefits or outcomes
- Quadrant 3: a graphic or pictorial representation of the problem, project, relevant data, outcomes, etc.
- Quadrant 4: a timeline

The amount of the funding requested (or a range of funding) fits best in quadrant 1 or 4.

Ultimately, you and your development officer may present the quad chart to the benefactor, or its contents might be incorporated into a longer, formal proposal. Regardless, the exercise will be invaluable in organizing your thinking around what you need, why you need it, connecting your need to your vision, and ensuring you and your development officer have a common understanding.

It would be a mistake to assume that because you are an expert in your field you will easily prepare a philanthropic proposal. To the contrary, your expertise can be an impediment to an effective proposal. You have spent years becoming an expert and you will face a strong temptation to convey that expertise. However, there are two simple (and all too common), related errors you must avoid in preparing a proposal: making it too complicated and too long. Many a proposal has been turned down for lack of clarity, either because of its sheer length or the presence of convoluted or complicated content.

The most effective way to prepare an effective proposal is to disengage from your "expert" self—something easier said than done—and put yourself in the shoes of the philanthropist, who may not have your knowledge in the content area.

Your proposal should convey a simple and succinct message, and in basic terms. By simple, we mean it should connect the dots between your interests, what you propose as a solution, and the impact of the solution (this is also why the quad chart is an effective tool to assist you). It may be appropriate to include some statistics to establish credibility and support your position, but they should be used sparingly. Philanthropists face real-world problems they want to solve. Toward this end, stories about tangible situations and people that clearly define the impact are a much-preferred method to convey meaning and results than are multiple statistics.

It can be hard to shape an important idea in a few words. Yet this is definitely a time to adhere to the adage, "less is more." Choose your words wisely. Use plain language, not jargon or heavily scientific verbiage, to create well-constructed, clear statements that will resonate with the reader. Using and repeating a memorable "tag line" provides the decision-maker a phrase that can be easily retained and conveyed to other individuals or groups.

Relatedly, we strongly recommend you spend some time early in your leadership tenure developing your "elevator speech" [4]. If you're not familiar with this term, it suggests you have about as much time to convey a meaningful idea as it takes to travel between a few floors in a building elevator (roughly 30–60 s). Remember, to maximize effectiveness, the pitch should be simple, direct, and vibrant, with a well-constructed hook ("tag line") that will stick in the listener's mind. Once you have your elevator speech drafted, practice saying it, and then practice some more. Share it with a mentor and/or your development officer for their input. You want to be ready to deliver it quickly and genuinely when the opportunity presents.

One basic framework to consider for crafting an effective elevator speech (or as another approach to developing a proposal) is to answer three simple questions: What? So What? Now What? The "What" answer provides the bottom-line issue, clearly and succinctly. Answering the "So what" targets why your "What" is important and outlines the intended outcomes, and the "Now What" answers what the listener can do to help.

For example, you are the chair of a Department of Dermatology that was recently established at your academic medical center. Dermatology services in your region are limited, and your department has the potential to expand rapidly. You would really like to recruit someone to your team with expertise in performing a certain type of surgery. In meeting a potential donor, you might share:

- (What?) *Our new department is growing fast, and I believe we can fill a significant void for services that has been needed in the community for a long time. We are seeing a lot of patients with skin cancer, which is the most common cancer in the United States. Two types in particular affect more than three million people each year.*[3]
- (So What?) *If we could recruit a dermatologist who specializes in the surgical technique to treat these forms of cancer, it would provide a much-needed form of care for people in our community, significantly increase our research in this area, and help to propel our program toward national prominence.*
- (Now What?) *With your investment to establish an endowed position in the department, I have no doubt we could recruit someone with a national reputation to our department. Would you be interested in scheduling a meeting with me and our development officer to talk further about this?*

An Investment, Not an Ask

Benefactors want to see their dollars used to transform the world and have a strong desire to feel part of something important. What better place to do that than in an academic medical center? Keep this in mind as you prepare your proposal and elevator speech. Namely, you are *not asking for a gift.*

Let's unpack this concept. First, you are not really asking so much as *inviting* the donor to join you in addressing an important undertaking. Secondly, you're not inviting them to make a gift, rather you're inviting them to make an *investment*, which

---

[3] American Academy of Dermatology Association (https://www.aad.org/media/stats-skin-cancer).

implies the donor has shared interest in (1) the initiative's success, (2) making a long-term commitment, and (3) like any investment, having an expectation of return.

From this perspective we believe, at its core, philanthropy is far more about relationships than money. "Philanthropic relationships" are partnerships with people who want to see you succeed and want be part of that accomplishment. It just so happens that they have the resources to assist in achieving that success.

Attaining this partnership may mean spending time learning about the benefactor, their goals, and aspirations. It may mean engaging in some appropriate self-disclosure. For example, benefactors may want to know about your career development, where you were educated, your leadership philosophy, etc. It may mean continually following-up with a benefactor. Immediately after an investment, this will take the form of an appropriate "thank you" to the benefactor. Ongoing relationship building may include subsequent communication (in writing or in person), periodic updates or reports (particularly on project progress or outcomes), invitations to future gatherings, a variety of forms of acknowledgement (assuming the benefactor consents), and future meetings to convey new opportunities. You're asking benefactors to invest in you, both personally and financially, and you should reciprocate by engaging them (to the extent they wish to be involved). In the parlance of development, this ongoing donor engagement is referred to as "stewardship."

It is certainly true that further investments sometimes result from effective stewardship. However, the primary purpose of stewardship is the ongoing expression of gratitude by forming and expanding genuine and meaningful relationships with donors, inviting them to participate in the "life" of your unit, and to see the "fruits" of their investment. Stewardship is not done simply so you can ask for another investment later.

We've commented a lot on the value of forming authentic relationships with donors, but to be maximally effective at philanthropy you also need to cultivate a solid relationship with your development officer. Get to know them on a personal level, spend time to learn about their style and approach, and work together to develop a strategy and shared approach. This relationship will do best if there is a solid level of trust between the two of you. Educate them about yourself and your unit (its history, vision, needs, key figures, relationship to the larger institution, etc.). The most effective, long-term philanthropic endeavors usually involve a three-way collaborative relationship among the leader, the development officer, and the benefactor(s).

The Process

There's no one best process for addressing philanthropy. As you and your development officer get to know one another, you will collectively develop your own preferred approach and process. To be clear, as leader you will not, or should not, be involved in every funding solicitation. Rather, the development officer, in partnership with you, is working to identify and engage a wide range of potential donors on a continuum, from wanting to learn more about your unit and its vision and goals, to those having a strong desire (or plan) to invest. When and how you're asked to engage with donors may be determined by the purpose of the engagement, the amount of a potential request, and the wishes of the donor.

Sometimes, you'll participate early in the process and provide a macro-level view of the situation. Other times, you'll be asked to participate in a solicitation meeting to represent your unit and convey to the donor the importance of their potential investment. Occasionally, you will be the first point of contact, such as if you know the benefactor or they are familiar with your work or unit. In these cases, it will be important for you to connect your development officer fairly quickly with the donor, to initiate the formal process for current and future gift giving.

Understand that as an emerging leader you represent not only your unit, but you serve as an ambassador for the larger academic medical center. Imagine being asked to fly hours from home to attend a donor event and being given only a few minutes to speak about your unit or initiative(s). This will happen, and at first it may seem like an ineffective use of your time. But it's important to recognize that your initiative may be one component of a larger gift that your institution is working toward, and it is thus equally important to recognize where you fit into the bigger picture. It may also be that your presentation is just the first of what will become increasingly longer and more detailed ones, as your development officer works through a larger group of potential donors to identify a single benefactor who resonates with your needs and interests.

We offer one important caution as it pertains to any process you and your development officer arrive upon. Not grasping the relational aspect of philanthropy as discussed above may cause you to fall prey to the temptation that, as the leader, you should be used as "the closer." By this we mean that you fall prey to the assumption that the development officer lines everything up with a potential benefactor, so you only have to go to one meeting and finish the donor agreement. In our experience, this is an ineffective (although unfortunately, not infrequently used) approach to philanthropy.

Regardless of the exact steps of the process, the last step is the most important, and no, the last step is not getting the money. The last step is appropriately saying "thank you." As a general rule of thumb, the scale of the thank you should match the magnitude of the gift. In other words, hosting a large reception for the donor and their extended family for a $3,000 expendable scholarship gift is probably excessive, but it might be very appropriate when recognizing the creation of a million dollar, named, endowed professorship.

In addition, a thank you is both a one-time event and an ongoing occurrence. As noted above, stewardship often takes the form of continual communication about the unit, invitations to events, annual acknowledgements, etc. The acknowledgement strategy should present a genuine conveyance of gratitude, which can sometimes turn the closure of one gift into the beginning of the next gift.

Philanthropists and Elected and Appointed Officials

It is very likely that in addition to engaging benefactors, as a new leader you're also going to encounter elected and appointed officials. These individuals are often state legislators, city council persons, and members of the university governing boards (e.g., members of the Board of Regents, or Board of Trustees).

We bring this to your attention as we believe philanthropists and governing officials have several things in common. Both control large financial resources, have significant problems they need/want to solve, and can greatly influence the trajectory of the academic medical center. Most emerging leaders have very little experience interacting with either of these groups.

We offer that the general principles for working with philanthropists can be equally well applied to working with elected and appointed officials. Like philanthropists, governing officials typically prefer straightforward and direct solutions to clear problems. And they want information about the impact that funding (or a policy) will have on your unit's goals, mission, or ability to achieve a desired outcome. Thus, the principles for preparing a benefactor proposal also apply when making a request of a governing official (or agency) or providing legislative testimony. Keep your remarks concise, use lay language, use statistics sparingly, and employ the use of stories about real situations and people. And as always, clearly define the impact a funding or policy decision would make.

Concluding Thoughts

We started this chapter by saying that leaders new to philanthropy may not like asking people for money. We hope this chapter has broadened your perspective on fundraising and increased your interest in participating in what can be a very exciting and personally meaningful aspect of your leadership role. Remember, whether working with philanthropists or governing officials, you will be more successful if you plan by putting yourself in their shoes. Provide them with the information, clarity, and outcomes they need, so you can help them to help you most effectively.

How Do I Get Started?

Philanthropy is a necessary component of higher education, and thus an element of the leader's job, at any level. To get started, find out who is your unit's development officer and begin building a relationship with that person. Learn how the development process works at your institution. Tap into your alumni base and have a clear strategy for communication with them. Lastly, have patience. Rome was not built in a day. Same with your philanthropic goals.

Coaching questions to ask yourself:
- How has my unit been doing with fundraising prior to my arrival as leader?
- What needs to be sustained, changed, jettisoned, or enhanced with my unit's fundraising strategy?
- Who do I know that is good at fundraising, and what can I learn from them?
- What are my hesitations about asking a donor for money? What is getting in the way of me performing better at fundraising?
- What would be different for my unit if I were better informed, prepared, and confident in fundraising?

Curious to learn more?
1. Doyle A. January 27, 2021. How to Create an Elevator Pitch With Examples: How to Write a Perfect Elevator Speech. Available at https://www.thebalancecareers.com/elevator-speech-examples-and-writing-tips-2061976
2. Eikenberry AM. 2009. Giving Circles: Philanthropy, Voluntary Association, and Democracy. Indiana University Press, Bloomington, IN
3. Thelin JR, Trollinger RW. 2014. Philanthropy and American Higher Education. Palgrave MacMillan, a division of Macmillan Publishers Ltd., England
4. Greer L, Kostoff L. 2020. Philanthropy Revolution: How to Inspire Donors, Build Relationships and Make a Difference. Harper Collins.
5. Perry R, Schreifels J. 2020. It's Not Just About the Money: How to Build Authentic Donor Relationships 2nd Ed. Independently Published.
6. Worth MJ, Lambert MT. 2019. Advancing Higher Education: New Strategies for Fund Raising, Philanthropy and Engagement. Rowman and Littlefield, Lanham, MD.

References

1. The Greatest Wealth Transfer in History: What's Happening and What are the Implications. Available at https://www.forbes.com/sites/markhall/2019/11/11/the-greatest-wealth-transfer-in-history-whats-happening-and-what-are-the-implications/?sh=2d38 32f94090
2. Charitable giving to U.S. colleges and universities reached $49.50 billion, Virtually Unchanged from Last Fiscal Year 2021. Available at https://www.case.org/resources/charitable-giving-us-colleges-and-universities-reached-4950-billion-virtually-unchanged
3. Project and Award Quad Chart Guidelines. Available at https://www.hsrd.research.va.gov/funding/quad_charts.cfm
4. Doyle A. January 27, 2021. How to Create an Elevator Pitch With Examples: How to Write a Perfect Elevator Speech. Available at https://www.thebalancecareers.com/elevator-speech-examples-and-writing-tips-2061976.

Accreditation: The Regulatory Lifeblood of the Academic Medical Center

15

If you've been around the academic medical center for any length of time, you're likely familiar with the accreditation process. We say "familiar" because many new leaders may be just that, generally aware, but having never actually participated in, much less led a formal process. Whether clinical, educational, or research related, a new leader will quickly come to appreciate that accreditation is the regulatory lifeblood of the academic medical center.

Accreditation intersects with virtually all missions of the academic medical center. For example, there are accrediting agencies for the clinical (patient care) mission [1], the research mission, [2] and the education mission [3]. With respect to the latter, there are both institutional or regional accreditation agencies (for the entire university), and specialized or programmatic accreditation agencies for each of the specific entry-level health professions, as well as graduate medical education (residency and fellowship programs) [4].

Since educating the next generation of health care professionals is a vital element of the academic medical center's mission, the examples we use throughout the chapter focus on academic accreditation. Our goal is to provide generalizable information on the purpose and process of all types of accreditation, providing what we hope are helpful insights for the new leader as they assume accreditation responsibility.

All types of accreditation are voluntary, non-governmental, peer review processes, although accreditation may be required to obtain certain governmental benefits or participate in certain federal programs [5]. Government agencies (e.g., Department of Education, Centers for Medicare & Medicaid Services) recognize the accreditation agencies as reliable organizations capable of determining quality through their standards and review processes, and thus accept or sanction their outcomes [6]. Accreditation processes generally consists of the initial application and review, followed by intermittent reporting and ongoing cycles of review.[1]

---

[1] The length of the accreditation cycle varies by the type of organization, the accreditation agency, and the results of the review, but is usually multiple years.

© The Author(s), under exclusive license to Springer Nature Switzerland AG 2022
K. P. Meyer, R. Kramer, *Taking the Lead*,
https://doi.org/10.1007/978-3-031-16711-9_15

A given periodic "review" usually consists of three parts: (1) the submission of the self-study prepared by the unit, (2) the site-visit, a few months after the submission of the self-study, conducted by a team of volunteer, accreditation agency trained independent reviewers,[2] and (3) the decision made by the accreditation agency commissioners, which follows the site visit and can also take a period of months.

Purposes of Accreditation

As we noted, accreditation is both a voluntary and necessary process. Depending on the type of unit being accredited, accreditation establishes the eligibility for academic institution to award degrees, for graduates to take licensure and certification examinations, for universities and students to obtain federal and state grants and loans, and for receiving some forms of healthcare reimbursement. Accreditation processes typically combine self and peer assessment, thus serving as a form of self-governance.

Accreditation standards establish a base-line level of expectation for the unit or organization. In doing so, accreditation safeguards the interests of the public. That is, it enables the public (be they patients, students, or research subjects) to know that a given organization has met the standards and regulations established by a recognized, external organization (the accrediting body), and is following industry identified and sanctioned best practices.

As noted above, because a given unit (hospital, college, institutional review board, etc.) undergoes accreditation on a periodic cycle, it is not uncommon that accreditation is viewed as an episodic event.[3] In this regard, accreditation is an intermittent *quality control measure*, the results of which represent the unit's performance at a point in time.

However, accreditation is also an ongoing process. Units are required to stay abreast of changes in standards, and as necessary, establish new policies and procedures to implement these updates. Many agencies have intermittent reporting requirements, and units are also required to communicate with the accreditation agency in the event of any substantive change (e.g., requests to increase enrollment, or add a new satellite campus). Units collect and maintain data to demonstrate their continual compliance with standards during the interim between formal reviews. This data is also used in preparing the next self-study. All these ongoing activities are intended to facilitate the other primary purpose of accreditation, *continuous quality improvement*.

---

[2] The site visit team also reviews the self-study. Site visitors possess expertise in the respective profession (e.g., a physician member of an LCME review team) or related fields (e.g., an anatomist on an LCME review team).

[3] i.e., a "point in time" determination of the extent to which the unit or organization meets the published standards.

Accrediting Agencies and Accreditation Standards

It is not the purpose of this chapter to list *all* the relevant accreditation agencies typically encountered by the academic medical center. We do, however, recommend that one of your first tasks when you assume your new leadership role should be to learn which accrediting agency(ies) your unit engages. Next, find out the date for the submission of the next self-study, as well as the status of its preparation. If the self-study is due within the upcoming 12-month timeframe, particularly if has yet to be started, the preparation and submission of the self-study may literally be your only job for the first months of your tenure as leader.

With respect to the academic mission, your academic medical center, as an entity, will undergo "institutional" or "regional" accreditation by one of six accrediting organizations. Each are approved by the U.S. Department of Education and the Council for Higher Education Accreditation (CHEA) to accredit all degree-granting institutions of higher learning in various geographic locations [7].

In addition to being accredited as an institution of higher learning, each specific health profession education program (e.g., medicine, dentistry, physical therapy, nursing, etc.) also undergoes what is termed "specialized" or "programmatic" accreditation. Specialized accreditation agencies establish and review standards that are specific to a given program of study. Multiple accrediting agencies exist that offer programmatic accreditation [8]. Unlike regional accreditation, specialized accreditation is conducted by the same agency for the same types of programs regardless of geographic location. For example, the Liaison Committee on Medical Education (LCME) accredits all U.S. medical schools, and the Commission on Accreditation in Physical Therapy Education (CAPTE), accredits all U.S. physical therapy programs.

The healthcare delivery (patient care) mission is accredited by different agencies, perhaps the best known being the Joint Commission [7]. Another agency, the Association for the Accreditation of Human Research Protection Programs (AAHRPP) [8] accredits institutional review boards (IRB) to ensure investigator and institutional compliance with regulatory requirements for the protection of human subjects in research.

Simply put, accreditation is the process of determining the extent to which the unit meets or is compliant with published accreditation standards. The standards are essentially declarative statements of expectations. For new leaders, what is sometimes confusing is that the standards indicate the *what*, but not the *how* (more on this later). Most accreditation agencies will offer some form of guidance to assist you in gathering and providing information deemed indicative of demonstrating compliance.

At the very least, this guidance usually includes specifically defined terms which appear in the accreditation standards glossary.[4] Defining terms creates standardization

---

[4] For example, see the Liaison Committee on Medical Education (LCME) Function and Structure of a Medical School, Standards for Accreditation of Medical Education Programs Leading to the MD Degree. March 2022. Available at https://lcme.org/publications/#Standards.

across the organizations or units seeking accreditation and adds clarity for compliance. It probably goes without saying, but it is imperative that you read these definitions and not make assumptions about the meaning of even fairly common words. Other forms of guidance include lists of examples of evidence, or "interpretive guidelines" that provide further detail about the intent of the standard and suggest strategies to demonstrate compliance.

Beginning the Accreditation Review Process

Since accreditation is a voluntary process, it is the responsibility of the unit or organization to make a formal request to initiate an initial (first) accreditation process. Generally, an application or letter of intent accompanied by required fees initiates this first review process. Once "in the system" the unit will follow the procedural guidance offered by the accreditation agency, which may include the awarding or recognition of some form of "interim" status (e.g., candidacy, new program accreditation, etc.). For new health profession education programs seeking programmatic accreditation, awarding of this interim status allows the institution to enroll students. After the initial formal review process, assuming full accreditation is awarded, the unit will be placed on a regular cycle for review.

The first step in the formal review is preparing the self-study. Depending on the unit's experience with accreditation and familiarity with the standards, we recommend you begin to assemble your accreditation team 18–24 months before your self-study report is due. For example, you will want to begin sooner if you need to send members of your team to an accreditation workshop. These are programs often offered at professional meetings. It's impractical to send an entire team to an accreditation workshop. However, it can be useful to send two members, for both clarifying and remembering extensive information, as well as for beginning to formulate the self-study writing plan. Additionally, because accreditation is a high stakes endeavor, some institutions also choose to engage consultants, or colleagues from other units, to conduct "mock" site visits. If this is something you are thinking of doing, plan accordingly. The recommended length of the preparatory phase should afford adequate time to conduct such a review and have time to incorporate any recommended changes.

We mentioned an accreditation *team* because we believe accreditation achieves the best outcomes when approached as a "team sport." The sheer volume of data collection and assembly requires the expertise of many, and that expertise can also be used in writing sections of the narrative (self-study). Engaging a wide array of unit (and campus) members in the process will not only help tremendously with gathering and cataloging all the necessary supportive data, but it will also more importantly, begin the process of "socializing" the self-study report within your unit, so everyone has knowledge of its content. The key here is that the *unit* is accredited, not the *leader*, so site visitors often evaluate the extent to which the members of the unit know and "own" the self-study.

Depending on the size of your unit, everyone may be on the team, but for larger units you may choose to appoint a representative team to oversee the preparation of the self-study. It's generally pretty clear who these members should be. For example, in the case of programmatic accreditation for a health professions education program, those overseeing various functional areas (e.g., curriculum, student services, finance and administration, etc.) would be responsible to assemble data and write the corresponding draft sections (or provide content and consultation to those who write).

This not only spreads the workload, but it also ensures those with the most current and relevant information are writing the section pertinent to their expertise. We do also however, recommend appointing "co-chairs" to lead the team, including someone known for their attention to detail, and someone with effective organizational and writing skills to serve as the "editor." The editor's primary responsibility is to organize the self-study narrative, ensure it meets format and word count guidelines, and ensure it is written in a consistent "voice." As leader, you may choose to serve this editor role, but we strongly encourage you not to assume sole responsibility for writing the self-study.

The first step in writing the self-study (and preparing for the site visit) is for the team to familiarize themselves with the accreditation standards and accompanying guidance (this is one of the benefits of attending an accreditation workshop). We cannot stress this step enough. While we recognize this step is laborious, review the standards in their *totality* before beginning to gather substantive evidence and writing the self-study. Many standards overlap. In the end, it is possible to save a lot of time for the team in preparing the self-study, and for the site visitors in reading the self-study, by connecting the dots between standards. This is especially true when the same or similar evidence can be used to demonstrate compliance with more than one standard.

Keep in mind too that the accreditation agency staff is available to assist you. If you have not worked with these individuals, think of them as the equivalent of a grant program officer. They will typically not provide direct advice (i.e., they won't tell you what to do), but they are there to assist you in understanding the standards and the process and answering questions about either.

Writing the Self-Study

We alluded to this earlier, accreditation standards are typically not prescriptive. Although evidence must be provided to substantiate compliance, the accreditation body allows each institution to "write their own story." Your self-study story demonstrates how your institution or unit meets the standards. In other words, the self-study weaves together and highlights the unique aspects of *your* unit or organization (mission, vision, values, financial modeling, strategic plan, enrollment goals, new initiatives, physical space, equipment, etc.) to demonstrate how your organization meets the accreditation standards.

Demonstrating compliance may seem like a rather simple concept, just list the stuff that's asked for, right? As simple as this may seem, sometimes people struggle to determine exactly what constitutes "evidence," or how to demonstrate that the evidence, in fact, meets the standard. Our caution in this regard is that saying you did something is not the same as providing tangible evidence that substantiates you did what you said.

For example, in response to a standard about conducting ongoing program assessment and planning, you may cite as one form of evidence that the entire faculty reviewed the admission processes and criteria at a regularly scheduled, weekly faculty meeting. This would be a perfectly acceptable response to identify the *process* by which the decision was made, but it doesn't provide the evidence to *prove* the standard was met.

To do the latter would require formal, dated meeting minutes that cite the referenced discussion, the data or information reviewed, and any corresponding action taken (e.g., voting to continue with the current criteria or adding an additional criterion). And as it pertains to both process and compliance, you can't just create minutes for the *one* meeting that you cite, you would need to have minutes for every faculty meeting to demonstrate this was your "typical" process for faculty decision-making.

Take for example another common standard requiring the sponsoring institution (college or university in the case of academic programs) to provide a given program with sufficient financial resources to operate the program. A common piece of data (evidence) in support of compliance would be the program's annual budget. However, in and of itself, a budget document would be insufficient to demonstrate "sufficient financial support," without also including a contextual description of the type of budget process the institution uses, how the annual budget is determined, if there are opportunities (either through an annual planning process, or mid-year if a need arises) to modify the budget, how research indirect costs are shared with the unit, how new positions are approved, etc.

We've established that accreditation typically combines self and peer assessment for the purposes of quality control *and* continuous quality improvement. So, it's important that the self-study identifies your unit's strengths and areas for needed improvement. You don't have to go to great lengths to highlight needed improvements, but don't try to hide them either. Be honest. It is far better that *you* identify areas for needed improvement and begin the improvement process, than to wait and receive a formal citation. That's what a self-study is all about!

Relatedly, if the unit received a citation or was required to implement remedial actions following the last accreditation review, make sure you identify how the issue was successfully addressed in the interim. If changes were not made or were insufficient, own that too. Identify why it wasn't addressed (or addressed fully) and begin immediately to implement the necessary changes. Whether you identify a new area for needed improvement, or indicate insufficient improvement about a previous issue, you will have the interim time between the self-study submission and the site visit to at least demonstrate a concerted effort to address these concerns.

One last thing about preparing the self-study, there's no need to "recreate the wheel." For example, there's usually a section that asks you to identify organizational resources (for educational programs this could be physical plant, library, student services, IT, study space, etc.). Similar information is requested by virtually every accreditation body that accredits health profession education programs. It's very likely that at least a template of this "typically" required information is available through the vice chancellor of academic affairs, the accreditation and assessment office, or a similar department. A good source of this information can also be the institutional self-study prepared for regional accreditation. You may need to adjust the content to the unique format requested by your accreditation agency, or to your unit, but you shouldn't have to collect all of this information and build it from scratch.

Once the self-study is written, socialize the primary content with the members of the unit and anyone else who will be interviewed by the site visitors. As we noted, it is important that all relevant parties take ownership of the accreditation process, not just the unit leader. It's far more difficult to demonstrate the institution values accreditation if only the leader knows the material. Toward this end, we also recommend preparing an executive summary of the self-study to share with the institution's executive team and other stakeholders who may be less familiar with the unit, so they can speak in an informed fashion with the site visitors.

Hosting the Site Visit

A site visit follows the submission of the self-study, although this is often several months later. As noted above, members of the site visit team are typically volunteers with requisite expertise and experience. For specialized accreditation, they may be professionals and/or faculty who are or have served in leadership roles within higher education or the profession (often both).

The site visit interaction is formal and professional. To avoid a conflict of interest, keep it non-relational. By this we mean, the unit should be cooperative and welcoming, but the primary role in "hosting" the site visit team is preparing the schedule, providing space for the team to conduct their work, and ensuring timely access to information, as requested. Activities you might otherwise do in hosting visitors, such as making hotel accommodations, providing airport transport, and taking them to dinner, are not necessary (and may in fact be prohibited), so as to avoid a conflict of interest.

Make it a priority to check-in with the team routinely during their visit. If they discover perceived inconsistencies or gaps, they may request additional information or explanation. Do your best to attend to these requests, as if they can be effectively addressed in "real time," you may be able to avoid a later request for additional information or perhaps even a citation.

Put succinctly, the site visit is essentially an external audit, so the site visitors will employ a variety of "validation" techniques. Interestingly, many of these are similar methods to those used in qualitative research, such as:

- Verification: Direct review of a sample of the data cited in the self-study (e.g., policies and procedures, visual inspection of facilities, review of budget data, etc.)

- Member checking: Meeting with those who wrote the report or have direct knowledge and interaction with the people and processes cited in the self-study, to confirm the content and accuracy of the self-study.
- Triangulation: "Connecting the dots" between multiple sources of data, and multiple people with varied roles to both validate, and obtain a more comprehensive understanding of the self-study and its findings.

At the conclusion of the site visit, the team will likely conduct an "exit interview," with the principal members of the unit or institution. This is the opportunity for the site visit team to report their general summary findings and identify strengths, as well as concerns or areas for improvement. To be clear, at best the exit interview should be viewed as a preliminary report of findings. It *does not represent an accreditation decision*. Rather, the site visit team will prepare a formal report they submit to the accreditation body for review and action.

If concerns were raised during the visit that could not be address in real time, you will receive a formal letter outlining the concerns. This generally comes before the final review by the agency commissioners, in which case your unit will have the opportunity to refute or address the finding by providing additional clarifying information and documentation (and remediation strategies, if necessary). This step may mitigate further action on the part of the accreditation agency. But if the issue is significant, it may still result in a citation. This will then require an additional response, in which you will likely be asked to identify your remediation plan, including responsible parties, and a timeline. Periodic submission of documentation demonstrating progress in completing the remediation plan will also likely be necessary.

Formal review of site visit reports by agency commissioners may only occur at certain pre-determined meetings, so depending on the timing of your site visit, it may be several months before you receive a formal notification and determination of accreditation status. Actions range from awarding full accreditation for an entire cycle, to denying accreditation, to intermediate actions like probation. The latter is usually accompanied by initial and intermittent reporting requirements and a shorter cycle before the next review. Accreditation agencies have formal appeals processes, so appeal of a formal finding may be yet another opportunity for a unit to provide additional information and clarification.

A Final Tip on the Schedule for the Site Visit

Most often the site visit team will identify the title of the individuals they need to meet (CEO, Dean, etc.), or a description of the groups they need to meet (students, faculty, healthcare providers, etc.). With respect to groups of individuals, you have considerable latitude in determining the participants. While it happens infrequently, regrettably, we have seen instances in which one (or at most a small faction) of faculty members or health care providers attempt to "highjack" the accreditation process to force action on something they feel has not been adequately addressed by the unit. These individuals often contend their issue is uniformly held, more so than it truly is. And as a self-appointed spokesperson, think that by exposing what they believe to be the unit's "dirty laundry," the accreditation agency will somehow force the unit to address their concern or achieve their preferred result.

The problem with this should be evident. Most often, the one or few individuals who choose to do this typically do not represent the unit's majority view. The risk here is that it may be difficult for the site visitors to fully discern what is happening. At best, these actions may create unnecessary work for you as the leader, and the team that wrote the self-study, as you may be required to provide additional documentation or compliance reporting. And at worst, the result could be a less favorable accreditation outcome, such as citations or a shortened accreditation cycle. To add insult to injury, the institutional harm that is created can last beyond the perpetrator's time of employment. To reiterate, accreditation is an organizational-level compliance audit, it is not an individual grievance process. To conflate the two puts the organization at great risk.

Thus, when assembling the groups that will talk to the site visitors, choose wisely. It is fine to select individuals representing a broad range of roles and experiences, but you want individuals that will present the unit or organization in a positive light, or if there are issues, to accurately represent the steps the unit is taking to address them. To reiterate what we said above, this advice presumes that if you have areas for needed improvement, you have identified these and the accompanying steps for improvement in your self-study.[5]

The goal is to give an accurate and realistic accounting of your situation, not to "muzzle" anyone. But we recommend you select individuals who understand and embrace the overarching goal of achieving accreditation and avoid including disgruntled individuals who may have ulterior motives. If the latter must be included, make sure to put them in groups where their views may be appropriately challenged or "balanced" by the collective view of the majority.

Concluding Thoughts

As you enter the leadership arena in the academic medical center you will quickly learn of value of accreditation. And there is considerably more detail to learn about your specific accreditation situation. In this process of learning, you may hear some people comment that accreditation processes are burdensome. We consent that undergoing accreditation is hard, time-consuming work, and for those new to accreditation, it can even be daunting at times. But, in our opinion, one we hope you share, accreditation is not only valuable, but it should also be welcomed. Done well, accreditation can serve as a tremendous tool for open and transparent communication, innovation, and continuous quality improvement. As importantly, it upholds and celebrates the values of all academic medical centers, including transparency, excellence, teamwork, and accountability.

---

[5] Accordingly, do not attempt to hide problems from the accreditation site team, as it never ends well.

How Do I Get Started?

Accreditation is a complex, multi-dimensional process. The first time guiding it can seem daunting. However, with an eye on both quality preparation and an outstanding site visit, the process can be smooth and rewarding. Talk to others who have experience leading a unit's accreditation process. Ask to see examples of self-studies to glean good ones from poorly written ones. Be thoughtful in scheduling, assigning, and hosting the site visit. And lastly, consider scheduling a vacation for after the process is over. You will have earned it and will likely appreciate the timely break.

Coaching questions to ask yourself:

- Who do I respect that might share their experience and self-study with me?
- Who do I know for sure should be on my unit's self-study team, and who do I know for sure should not?
- What are my glaring weaknesses in leading this process, and who can help me compensate for these gaps?
- What do I need to learn right now?
- How can I mitigate uncertainties and minimize surprises during this process?
- If I discover areas for needed improvement, who can assist me in developing strategies and reasonable timelines?
- How will I take care of myself and support the care of the self-study team as we embark on this process?

Curious to learn more?

1. Frank, J.R., Taber, S., van Zanten, M. et al. The role of accreditation in twenty-first century health professions education: report of an International Consensus Group. *BMC Med Educ* 20, 305 (2020). https://doi.org/10.1186/s12909-020-02121-5
2. Phillips S.D., Kinser K (eds.). (2018). Accreditation on the Edge: Challenging Quality Assurance in Higher Education. Johns Hopkins University Press, Baltimore, MD. ISBN/DOI 978–1,421,425,443
3. Gaston, P.L. (2014) Higher Education Accreditation: How It's Changing, Why it Must. Stylus Publishing, Sterling, VA.
4. U.S. Department of Education. Accreditation in the U.S. Available at https://www2.ed.gov/admins/finaid/accred/accreditation.html
5. U.S. Department of Education. History and context of accreditation in the United States Available at https://www2.ed.gov/admins/finaid/accred/accreditation_pg2.html

References

1. https://bhmpc.com/calltoaction/accreditation-comparison-cta/Accreditation-Comparison-Tool.pdf.
2. https://www.aahrpp.org/.
3. Council for Higher Education Accreditation. Accreditation and Recognition. Available at: https://www.chea.org/chea-and-usde-recognized-accrediting-organizations.
4. Accreditation Council for Graduate Medical Education. Available at: https://www.acgme.org/.
5. Congressional Research Service. An Overview of Accreditation of Higher Education in the United States. Updated October 16, 2020. Available at: https://sgp.fas.org/crs/misc/R43826.pdf
6. Kelly M. Joint Commission 101: What is "Deemed Status" and Who Grants It? 2020, January 21. Available at https://home.akitabox.com/blog/deemed-status-and-joint-commission.
7. The Joint Commission. Available at https://www.jointcommission.org/.
8. Association for the Accreditation of Human Research Protection Programs, Inc. Available at: http://www.aahrpp.org/.
9. Council for Higher Education Accreditation (CHEA). Regional Accrediting Organizations. Available at: https://www.chea.org/regional-accrediting-organizations-accreditor-type#:~:text=The%20United%20States%20is%20divided,commissions%20operate%20in%20these%20regions.
10. Colleges and Degrees. Healthcare and Accreditation. Available at: https://www.collegesand-degrees.com/accreditation/healthcare-accreditation.

Part IV

Leadership Challenges and Challenges to Leadership

Leading Change in the Academic Medical Center

16

Change is a constant in every industry, and the academic medical center is no exception. For starters, change occurs each year in the life of the academic medical center as new students and residents begin their respective educational journeys. Other changes take many forms, from quality improvement changes to advance clinical care, to changes in policies and procedures which maintain a variety of regulatory compliance requirements, to the development of new research discoveries, and the addition or expansion of education and clinical programs. Literally, not a day goes by that does not see some change.

We stated from the beginning that we did not intend to summarize the existing literature on leadership, which is replete with information on change management and leaders as change agents. Yet, knowing that change is both continuous and necessary for the survival of academic medical centers, we did think it was important to highlight some of its unique features in this environment to promote your skills as an effective, thriving change agent.

A "Systems" Perspective on Change

To understand how to effectively implement change in your academic medical center, you first need to understand the big picture. The fundamental and primary place we recommend you begin before starting any change process is to recognize that academic medical centers are complex systems. And the humans working in this environment also function in systems. As Donella Meadows, professor, scientist, and educator states [1]:

> A system isn't just any old collection of things. A system is an interconnected set of elements that is coherently organized in a way that achieves something (p. 11).

Meadows goes on the clarify that, "a system must consist of three kinds of things: *elements*, *interconnections*, and a *function or purpose* [2]".

© The Author(s), under exclusive license to Springer Nature Switzerland AG 2022   149
K. P. Meyer, R. Kramer, *Taking the Lead*,
https://doi.org/10.1007/978-3-031-16711-9_16

Consider the academic medical center as a system. The *elements* include the many colleges, departments, divisions or sections, and programs that make up the entity, as well as the hospital, clinics, labs, and administrative sites. They are *interconnected* through the organizational chart and the complex network of reporting assignments, budgets, relationship of academic departments and the hospital(s), interdisciplinary research, outpatient clinics, multiple campus sites, and the list goes on.

The *function* of this system is to provide education (training the next generation of healthcare providers), clinical care (both routine and complex), research (advancing knowledge in health and healthcare to ultimately improve the public's health), and community engagement (increasing access to care and advancing the communities' health). In its entirety, this "system" we call the academic medical center is designed to serve the greater good.

Why be aware of all this? Any change made to one aspect of a system has a radiating effect on the other parts of the system. If you make a change that targets an *element* in the system, for example create a new research center, it has impacts on administrative oversite, reporting, and budgeting – the interconnections in the system. Change an aspect of *interconnections*, for example implementing a new electronic medical record system, and essentially all elements of the organization must adapt to it. Lastly, if you make a change to the *purpose*, for example add a new campus location, you have a new identity that drastically changes the system's elements and interconnections.

Maintaining a systems perspective will keep you mindful of the impacts change has on every aspect of the academic medical center. It will help with effective planning, implementation, and finding effective strategies to mitigate challenges or resistance to change.

Change as "Perturbation"

Since we're writing about change in academic medical centers, we thought it would be useful to use a clinical metaphor as a model for change. Physical therapists (Kyle's profession) refer to a physical external force that destabilizes a current state of equilibrium as a "perturbation" (from the base work perturb). For example, someone running by to catch the bus accidently bumps into you, destabilizing your equilibrium and causing you to fall. In this example, your state of equilibrium is the degree of "certainty or stability" you *were* experiencing before being bumped. If the force exerted by the other person (the perturbation) is of sufficient strength to overcome the counterforce (your stable equilibrium), you will move (fall).

To illustrate this concept, refer to the red ball in Fig. 16.1a. The ball is experiencing stable equilibrium, "protected" in the well called the "current state." To initiate change, the ball must first be forced out of that well (perturbed), by physically pushing it out of the well and then "up the hill" (Fig. 16.1b). With sufficient external force, the ball will eventually "make if over the hump" and into a different well called the "new normal," in which it will regain a state of equilibrium (Fig. 16.1c).

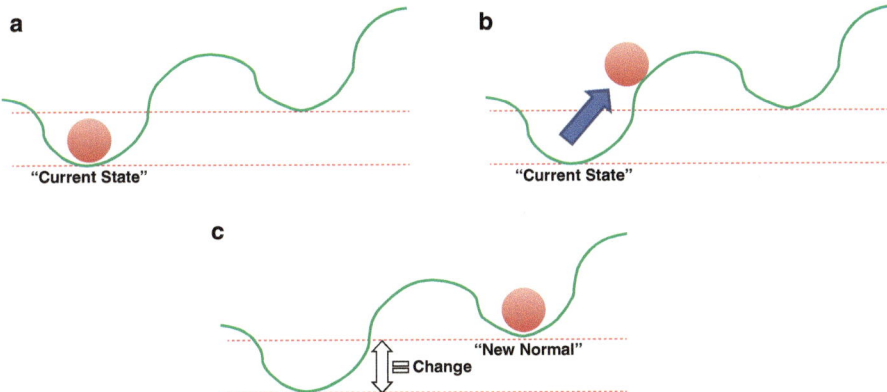

Fig. 16.1 Conceptual model of change. (**a**) Current or "stable" state of equilibrium. (**b**) External force required to initiate movement out of "stable" state. (**c**) The difference between the intial and new states of equilibrium represents change

These diagrams illustrate several general truths about change. First, they acknowledge the value of the state of equilibrium (certainty). Secondly, they demonstrate that work (force) is required to achieve change (i.e., change is not a "downhill phenomenon"). Thirdly, we can define the degree of change as the difference between a former and a new state of equilibrium. Fourth, more force (energy) is required at the beginning of the process to move the ball out of its current state of equilibrium, and if steady force is not continually applied when the ball is on the "uphill" climb it will readily return to its former state.

But once the ball is *just* over the top of the hill, the amount of external force can decrease (one final push may be required at the top to get the ball "over the hump"), as momentum takes over and carries the ball (change) into the new well. This series of illustrations illuminates the truths about the process of change, and it clarifies the expression you may hear leaders say about initiating change… *"It feels like I'm pushing a boulder uphill."* Which is also why it's so important to gain early adopters (see Chap. 9)—you need others to help push!

Time to Change and Time for Adapting to Change

There's no "rule of thumb" for when to introduce a change initiative. While the academic medical center as an organization is in constant change, we believe the people working in them need to be afforded time to prepare for and adapt to change. We recommend, when possible, spending much more time discussing the need for, and the *possibility* of, future change with those it will affect before ever initiating an actual change initiative.

After the change has occurred people also need time to adapt to whatever situation resulted from the change. Refer again to Fig. 16.1c. You can envision the ball rocking back and forth as it enters the new well before finally "coming to rest." This illustrates the point that humans (and systems) need time to adapt (to settle into the certainty of the "new state" well), at least for a brief period. New patterns and practices resulting from the change need time to be analyzed, improved, and smoothed out.

While change is a *constant* phenomenon in academic medical centers, it is hard for systems and people to endure change *constantly*. A leader who introduces continuous change initiatives and fails to recognize the need for periods of equilibrium (adaption and a return to some "certainty"), will likely be met with increasing resistance to subsequent change efforts as their followers experience a phenomenon referred to as "change fatigue" [3].

While there are some typical reasons people resist change (e.g., fear, inertia), we have observed situations that could be misinterpreted as resistance to change yet might more accurately can be categorized as the inadvertent effects of poor timing for introducing change. People seem less likely to embrace a change initiative, or perhaps have less capacity for change, if there is a high degree of "environmental uncertainty," whether national, local, or personal levels of insecurity. For example, political unrest, economic downturns, personal illness, or other family events can spark change resistance. It's almost as if people are saying to themselves, "The only thing I have control of is my work, so I'm going to hunker down and maintain what I know!" Conversely, when things seem to be going well (or better) in the national, local, or personal environment, we find people to be more amenable to considering workplace change.

Another thing we've noticed about people's willingness to consider change is how well the proposed change matches their "time horizon." As the leader, your role as visionary and chief strategist includes you regularly considering the needs and opportunities of your organization as far as 3–5 years into the future. A department chair or program director, however, may have a time horizon of 1–3 years, as they consider such questions as, what new service needs to be developed? Who needs to be recruited and hired? Should we conduct a major revision of the curriculum? On the other hand, a faculty member who needs to get their course developed and approved by the curriculum committee and then uploaded to the learning management system, is typically concerned with a time horizon of the academic year or maybe only the semester. Thus, they may have a 6 month to 1-year time horizon. The point is, if as the leader you introduce a change you know will benefit the unit in 3 years, you may not perceive a lot of initial support from faculty who are focusing their time and energy on meeting the responsibilities of the current semester.

We realize it's nearly impossible for you, as leader, to time the introduction of a new change initiative for when there is high environmental certainty (if there even is such a thing), or to alter the time horizon of those you lead. Rather, we share these observations to elevate them in your awareness, both in considering how you might modify the timing of an introduced change, and also to help you recognize that the need (or timing) for change can be viewed differently by individuals or subgroups, based on their roles in the unit.

Practical Recommendations for Leading Change in the Academic Medical Center

Over the years, we have had discussions about change with people from other industries outside of academia and healthcare. They are often surprised that change is such a *process* (perhaps, more accurately, such a long process) in the academic medical center. In their business, change is the result of the CEO or Board of Directors saying a change is needed, introducing it, and expecting everyone to comply in a given timeframe. As noted in Chap. 2 (The Milieu of the Academic Medical Center), reliance on shared governance, broad stakeholder input, and "egalitarian" decision-making does not equate to the system supporting a "top down" change directive. Introducing and guiding change in an academic medical center is more likely to succeed with a transparent and evidenced-based process. Change initiatives have better outcomes when they include several clearly defined elements, including (1) a well-articulated rationale or purpose, (2) a well-defined process for preparing for and implementing the change, (3) clear timelines with benchmarks, and (4) the identification (or assignment) of responsible and accountable individuals guiding and supporting the process.

With respect to the purpose or rationale for change, we recommend, especially early in your tenure as new leader, that you explicitly identify when the proposed change is in response to an "external force." If you can identify the need to change as a response to a newly implemented policy, compliance requirement, funding opportunity, business contract, etc., change may be easier to introduce and with less resistance, as the need to change is tangible and perhaps even "outside your hands."

Similarly, even if *you* are the initiator of the change, we would still recommend connecting the need to an external or environmental necessity. For example, aspirational goals, national developments in health professions education, innovations at other universities, or predicted future trends in healthcare are all excellent reasons for change.

From a process perspective, using "trial balloons" or "pilot programs" as a component of the change initiative allows for refinement, people seeing tangible benefits, and ultimately broader adoption of the change initiative. Additionally, engaging and celebrating early adopters (see Chap. 9) is a key to promoting change, as others will witness public recognition and reward for those supporting the change – influencing broader participation.

As we noted earlier, change in academic medical centers is fairly constant, in part because most change is iterative. Inviting feedback, thoughtfully considering input, and making necessary modifications can also dramatically improve adoption and trust. Refer to the eight strategies to increase your success in incremental pluralism, outlined in Chap. 2, as they represent very practical steps for initiating and achieving successful change initiatives in the academic medical center.

Everyone Is a Change Agent

We discussed earlier that a leader's primary responsibility is to provide a compelling vision. A compelling vision mobilizes people to get great things done because everyone assumes ownership and accountability for the outcome of the vision. A great vision is essentially an invitation to change – to collectively engage in the work that will catalyze the organization to achieve its preferred future.

In detailing the evolution of the Joint Special Operations Task Force, General Stanley McChrystal et al. [4], summarized two key elements that allow for any organization to maximize its ability to meet its mission and achieve its vision. The first is that the members of the organization must have a "shared consciousness." McChrystal and his coauthors state,

> We wanted to fuse generalized awareness with specialized expertise. Our entire force needed to share a fundamental, holistic understanding of the operating environment and of our own organization, and we also needed to preserve each team's distinct skill sets. We dubbed this goal – this state of emergent, adaptive, organizational intelligence – *shared consciousness*, and it became the cornerstone of our transformation [5] (italics added).

The second, McChrystal et al., describe as "empowered execution." This is the notion that the person closest to the decision should be empowered to make it.

What does this mean for you as an academic medical center leader? Well, we hope it changes your view about change. Rather than thinking it is solely *your* responsibility to introduce and shepherd change initiatives, we offer that the role of the leader is to create an environment where each member of the unit comes to understand themselves as a change agent. To achieve this outcome, the leader must explicitly communicate to each member that understanding and fulfilling their prescribed role and responsibilities is critical to the success of the unit, but it is insufficient. To reach a level of excellence in achieving the unit's daily missions, and to ultimately reach the future preferred state, everyone must possess and embrace a clear, mutual understanding of the big picture.

Once that shared understanding is in place, each member must be given the opportunity and responsibility to execute their role as it pertains to achieving the mission and vision. However, it's possible that individual members of your unit could be very successful in their own right (as is often the case at academic medical centers) and contribute less to the overall success of the unit. That's why McChrystal et al., identify the unifying function of shared consciousness as the key to successful, empowered execution, noting,

> An organization should empower its people, but only *after* it has done the heavy lifting of creating shared consciousness (italics in the original) [6].

The idea of everyone in the organization understanding the bigger picture is perfectly illustrated in an experience one of the co-authors (Rob) had when he was hired by a university to create and launch a leadership center. The president of the university had painted a vision of where he wanted the university to go, and he wanted *all* employees to embrace and help the campus move toward that vision.

Hence, the primary goals of the center were to have (1) every employee (faculty, staff, and administrators) see that they were a leader, regardless of job title, and (2) every employee understand and embrace how their role fit into the accomplishment of the university's mission. Creating and implementing this organizational process of shared direction, alignment, and commitment [7] across the entire workforce was a massive change process, and the center was used to catalyze and energize it. Fast forward a decade and this university is one of the top academic institutions among its peers. This is not to say that the work of the leadership center was solely responsible for the change, but it was a key component of a larger vision the president held as he frequently and routinely communicated it to the campus community.

Closing Encouragement

There is no "sugar coating" it, change is hard work. And you will have your detractors. As we close this section on change in the academic medical center, we do so with what might be an obvious caution that, despite your best efforts to effectively introduce change and to help each member of your unit join you as their own change agent, you will no doubt experience resistance to change initiatives throughout your career. Even so, we want you to remain encouraged. If your vision is well thought out, inspirational, aspirational, and attainable—and your supervisor(s) support it, you should be courageous to work toward achieving it.

Your goal as the leader is to help everyone understand the need for and the value of change as it pertains to accomplishing the missions and achieving the vision. By carefully deploying the strategies noted above, we believe you can win over most of individuals who may initially oppose change. But for the few individuals that can't be won over or won't align with the vision, it is better, in our experience, if you engage in the ultimate change initiative by encouraging them to find a place in another unit or organization with a vision that more closely aligns with their needs.

How Do I Get Started?

This may sound campy, but change starts with you, as the leader. People can see through the veneer of false hope, so you must be fully committed to, and believe in the change you are leading. That alone takes energy, drive, dedication, and the willingness to deal with resistance, setbacks, and numerous days when you may want to give up. Despite the obstacles, one of the many joys of leadership is driving towards something that you can see that others may not yet, and helping their light bulbs come on to the value of the change.

Coaching questions to ask yourself:
- Why is this change important—to me? To the organization?
- How will the change impact the long-term outcomes for our unit?
- What do I need to do to fully understand how my unit/organization will respond before and during the change process?
- Who would be good early adopters?
- What supports do I need for myself to sustain my motivation during the ups and downs of this implementation?
- If I find myself feeling overwhelmed by the entirety of a change process, ask "what is just the next step in the process?" (As opposed to thinking about all that needs to be done.)

Curious to learn more?
1. Bridges, W. (2009). Managing Transitions: Making the Most of Change. Da Capo Lifelong Books; third edition.
2. Kaplan, G. S. (2018). Building a Culture of Transparency in Health Care. Harvard Business Review. https://hbr.org/2018/11/building-a-culture-of-transparency-in-health-care.
3. Kotter, J. P. (1996). Leading change. Harvard Business School Press.
4. Meadows, D. H. (2015). Thinking in Systems. Chelsea Green Publishing.
5. Oshry, B. (2007). Seeing Systems: Unlocking the Mysteries of Organizational Life. Berrett-Koehler.
6. Senge, P. (2006). The Fifth Discipline: The Art & Practice of The Learning Organization. Doubleday.

References

1. Meadows DH. Thinking in systems. Chelsea Green Publishing; 2015.
2. Ibid, p. 11.
3. National Institute for Children's Health Quality, How to Cope with Change Fatigue. Available at: https://www.nichq.org/insight/how-cope-change-fatigue
4. McChrystal S, Collins T, Silverman D, Fussell C. Team of teams: new rules of engagement for a complex world. New York, NY: Penguin Random House; 2015.
5. Ibid, p. 153.
6. Ibid, p. 244.
7. McCauley C. Making leadership happen. Center for Creative Leadership; 2014. https://www.ccl.org/articles/leading-effectively-articles/make-leadership-happen-with-dac-framework/.

Leading Conflict Resolution

17

If you haven't yet figured it out up to this point, leading people comes with great rewards and many great challenges. The sheer size and scope of academic medical centers, not to mention sometimes competing interests, make it almost inevitable that you will encounter periodic conflict. This chapter presents important concepts and strategies to assist you in becoming more effective at conflict resolution, particularly in having the difficult conversations often accompanying conflict resolution. We also comment briefly on the related activities of negotiation and mediation, noting some parallels between these processes and conflict resolution, as well as the application of a few conflict resolution techniques to these equally important areas.

General Principles of Conflict Resolution

Conflict resolution is a general term defined as the "informal or formal process that two or more parties use to find a peaceful solution to their dispute." [1, 2] Two related processes or "forms" of conflict resolution include negotiation and mediation, although it should be noted that not all negotiation involves conflict. Collectively these processes share some commonalities in that they all:

1. Involve interactions between at least two people, albeit, often with different goals and perspectives.
2. Can be administered in both formal and informal manners.
3. Are commonly carried out in a face-to-face interaction (when possible).
4. Can evoke strong emotional reactions—that may or may not visibly emerge during or outside of the process.

More specifically, negotiation involves the process of discovery and discussion, the goal of which is to reach a mutually agreed upon decision (i.e., agreement). In addition to exploring mutually beneficial outcomes, the process should also include identifying the best and most plausible alternatives if a jointly approved agreement cannot be reached. [3] Negotiations occur formally or informally over any number of topics or issues. In the academic medical center, the "formal" process of negotiation most routinely and predictably concerns resources and workload (negotiating salary, start-up packages, bonuses, space, distribution of indirect cost returns, FTE distribution, etc.). A negotiation can also involve many people, such as a team assembled from across the academic medical center to negotiate a property acquisition. For the emerging leader, most negotiations will likely involve two people, you and the person with whom you are negotiating.

Mediation, on the other hand, involves at least three people, as it is a dispute resolution or arbitration process that engages an "objective" third party. The role of the mediator is not to determine or prescribe an outcome. Rather, the mediator guides the disputants in discovering and expressing their positions and interests to develop a resolution [1, 3]. Mediation can take the form of formal and informal processes. Leaders in academic medical centers may serve in the "informal" role of mediator, such as in helping to resolve disputes between members of a team or unit.

Additionally, many academic medical centers have an Ombuds Office. In as much as it is a recognized option for mediation, the process led by an ombudsperson tends to be "semi-formal," but an ombudsperson typically does not have decision-making or disciplinary authority. Rather, they work with disputants to solve their differences without initiating formal dispute resolution processes available in the academic medical center.

Lastly, the academic medical center has committees and offices (e.g., Title IX, grievance committee, professional conduct committee, etc.) that adjudicate formal grievances, complaints, or disciplinary actions using established procedures. Depending on the nature of the grievance and the personnel involved, the process may be administered by the Human Resources department or the Faculty Senate, among others. Formal processes involving students or residents are generally adjudicated by college-level committees.

Fundamental Elements of Conflict Resolution

As a general rule of thumb, conflict resolution, and the associated processes of negotiation and mediation could all be considered relatively "high risk." That is, the outcomes are very important to both parties, and considerable care and caution should be exercised to obtain a favorable outcome. As such, we think it is crucial for the emerging leader to be competent navigating these activities effectively and successfully. To begin, let's consider several important elements associated with these processes from a broad perspective.

Content or Relationship?

Conflict resolution typically involves having difficult conversations. When preparing, a first question you might ask yourself is, which should guide my role in this situation, focusing on the content (issue) or on the person (relationship)? The answer of course is both.

As it pertains to content, a part of conflict resolution that can often be more challenging than people think is defining the *real* problem or issue. Content definitely matters, and this is a crucial step to get right. Spend a suitable amount of time with the involved parties, before and/or during the process, defining and clarifying the context and purpose of your meeting. It's also easier than you might think to get off track during these conversations. Consequently, returning to the clarified and agreed upon issue(s) and purpose can help the process stay focused and progress forward.

People and relationships, of course, matter as well, as these processes exist to help people come to a resolution. In many instances, the processes are carried out between individuals who either have had or need to continue an ongoing relationship. It is essential to recognize the dynamics between the parties, as well as understand which side of the power dynamic *you* sit. Ultimately, and assuming all parties will continue working together in the academic medical center, one important goal should be maintaining or even advancing the relationship while coming to a successful resolution.

Process

In utilizing the process effectively, the leader needs to understand the difference between positions and interests. This distinction was made by Roger Fisher and William Ury in their seminal book, "Getting to Yes: Negotiating Agreement without Giving In" [3]. The authors note, "your position is something you have decided upon. Your interests are what caused you to so decide." [4] In other words, "positions" tend to be more fixed, whereas "interests" can be varied and multiple. Fisher and Ury argue that negotiating around positions can create a zero-sum game in which there is a "winner" and a "loser." However, by focusing on interests (those conditions underlying one's position), the parties can identify and clarify shared conditions or benefits, and thus arrive at mutually acceptable, negotiated outcomes.

Toward this end, work to anticipate the needs of the other party and be alert for solutions that meet mutual interests. Try to utilize "yes, and" as opposed to "yes, but" language to create a conversation that is generative versus limiting. And use the best available, comprehensive, correct, and mutually agreed upon data to assist in identifying shared interests and guiding decision-making.

Lastly, clarify the "boundaries" for the parties involved, including yourself. Understand the limits or constraints each party must work within so as not to promote possible solutions that are beyond the capacity of one or both parties to achieve. Realistically evaluate your position, that is, neither over value your position nor prematurely compromise on your position. And do not overpromise. Overvaluing your position or over-promising will eventually betray the trust and create resentment by the other party or lead to regret for yourself.

Tenor and Language

During the process, pay close attention to your attitude and language. Despite good and popular advice, it is difficult to totally eliminate emotions from some processes. Do your best to control strong emotional responses when they begin to arise. In these moments, it can be effective to be self-disclosing, modeling healthy behavior to advance the process. For example, if you feel yourself getting defensive, you might pause the conversation and say, "I am feeling myself wanting to get self-defensive and would like to take a moment to refocus." Then concentrate on maintaining positive regard and exhibiting empathy, for example by saying, "I hear you and can see why that would be challenging for you."

Words should be chosen carefully. Try to avoid using "emotionally-laden" or accusatory words. Remain vigilant about providing concise and specific responses. Most processes are best served with clear and succinct communication. Toward this end, we encourage you to avoid prefacing and apologizing. People often do this unconsciously, in response to an anticipated emotional response on the part of the listener, as well as to increase the level of comfort between the participants. You may be inclined to say something, especially in difficult situations, to "soften the blow." As examples, saying the following at the start is *prefacing*: "I wish we didn't have to have this conversation and I hope we can get through it together." Saying the following after having shared something difficult is *apologizing*: "I can see you are unhappy with what I said, I just want to reiterate I am only trying to help…" These strategies, though perhaps well intentioned, often distract and weaken the process.

When engaged in difficult conversations, we also recommend avoiding the popular "sandwich" approach to giving feedback—placing "negative" feedback between two positives. This strategy, while intended to diminish the level of discomfort between participants, also tends to weaken the clarity and purpose of the message.

Lastly, pay close attention to the tone of your voice, including volume, pitch, inflection, and rate. [5] Be deliberate about employing these elements, as they can have as great an impact on the hearer (and their response) as the actual words you say. Also, be intentional about consciously monitoring the other party's response, as it provides data that can guide you in maintaining or changing the elements of your tone.

Conscious Listening

Despite our encouragement about what to say and how to speak, the primary skill for all these processes to work effectively is listening. Commit yourself to listen more than you talk (even if the other party talks a lot). And commit to consciously listen, which is the process of deliberately analyzing and deciphering what you hear *in the moment*. This involves not only hearing the words the other party is saying but interpreting the deeper point or meaning they are trying to convey. [6] Be alert, as well, to spatial relationships, body language, eye contact, silence, etc., as these "meta-communication" factors also convey important data about how the other person views the conversation or situation.

As you develop "working interpretations," of what is being shared, validate them with the other party to avoid misinterpretation. For example, if you perceive the other party is "shutting down," you might say, "I notice you are being very quiet. I wonder if this is a topic you would rather not discuss, or did I say something to offend you?" This communicates to the other party that you are in fact listening intently and invites a response that may assist in redirecting the conversation.

Alternatively, do not be afraid to express your own emotional responses. In handling an aggressive statement by the other party, a display of conscious listening might include, "Just now when you said, 'That's ridiculous,' your volume was raised, you leaned in, and you banged your hands on the table. It makes me feel like I am being bullied into supporting your opinion. I would suggest we start again."

Conscious listening is a tremendous skill that will allow you to build the relationship, reframe what you have heard, and derive creative solutions. It takes a commitment and considerable practice to both participate in a conversation and reflect on it *as it is occurring* (see Chap. 5, "Reflection in Action"). The good news is that conscious listening is a skill that can be (or should be) used in any conversation, not just in conflict resolution. We encourage you to practice this skill under "less stressful" conditions, such as with a mentor or trusted colleague, so it becomes more authentic and automatic when you need to employ it in real time.

Avoid Avoiding Difficult Conversations

Difficult conversations are in most respects, well, difficult. Like crisis management, difficult conversations should not be viewed as interactions the leader is forced to engage, nor something to be avoided. Rather, they are simply part of the role, and a necessary and productive part at that. If the leader wants to ensure the success of the vision, the organization, and its members, difficult conversations are a natural part of the process.

While not all difficult conversations involve disagreements, many do. Having a difficult conversation requires contemplation and preparation, but it can sometimes cause the leader to second guess whether to have the conversation. For example, the leader may ask themselves, "Do I have the ability (or right) to confront this member of my team?" and perhaps, "Is it worth it?" Ruminations may follow, such as "maybe it's just a personality difference," "maybe my concern is just a generational difference," "I'll watch a little while longer," or "first, I'll try to give the person some more guidance, or clearer instructions."

These examples of self-talk, while necessary, don't reflect the changes in behavior that likely need to be made. Consequently, while being contemplative is a valuable tool, be mindful not to let necessary reflection derail *actually* having the difficult conversation. Doing so can (quite literally) lead to years of problems for both the leader and the person(s) with whom the conversation should have occurred.

Steps for Having a Difficult Conversation

We recommend you follow a general format when having a difficult conversation, not as a "prescriptive" requirement, but rather to enhance the conversation's effectiveness by ensuring certain elements are consistently addressed. Following a format will also aid you in remembering the conversation in the event you choose (or need) to write a summary of the interaction.[1] As an example, the process below focuses on a performance feedback conversation between an assistant dean (AD) for clinical research and one of her clinical trials directors.

The Opening of the Meeting

- Thank the individual for joining the meeting and indicate the general reason you called the meeting. Avoid saying things like, "I suspect you know why you're here," or "I'm sure we both wish we weren't having this meeting."

  AD: *Thanks for taking a few minutes to meet. I want to discuss some concerns I have about a specific area of your performance."*

- Briefly review the relevant data. This could include the incumbent's rôle and relevant responsibilities, the basic "problem" or problematic behavior as understood at this point in time, as well as the parties involved. Be as specific as possible.

  AD: *"I have received four separate complaints over just the past months about some of your interactions with members of your clinical trial team."*

- Do not suggest motive or intent associated with the behavior, such as, "I think you just don't trust your research project manager to get the job done." Rather, indicate your (and others' as appropriate) perceptions resulting from the behavior.

  AD: *"It's concerning to have received so many complaints. My perception is that some members of your team are not responding favorably to your leadership, and I am concerned for you, your team, and the trial's sustained success."*

The Middle of the Meeting

- Clarify the facts and (if warranted) the need for any additional information. Invite the incumbent to explain their behavior and respond to your perceptions. The incumbent will generally want to be heard. And if listening consciously, the leader will better understand the incumbent's perspective.

  AD: *"I am curious to understand your perspective of how things are going with your clinical trial team, and how I can be of help with this situation."*

---

[1] Such notes may simply be for your file, or to create minutes to share with the other party. They may be necessary to document a formal disciplinary process. Check with your Human Resources Department for procedural guidance.

- Listen well. Thank the incumbent for their input and indicate what behavior(s) is of concern and why it is incompatible with the successful performance or the expectations of the role.

    AD: *"Thanks for sharing your observations. It sounds like a lot to manage. One thing you mentioned caught my attention. It appears your desire for multiple check-in's a day with the team is being received as micro-managing. That may be having a negative impact on your team's performance, as well as their perception of your leadership. We would prefer the issue not escalate.*

- If the incumbent is receptive, this may provide an opportunity to mutually explore solutions. If not, you can proceed to be more directive with your expectations.

The End of the Meeting

- Indicate it is your responsibility as the leader to provide feedback.
- Indicate your expectation for improved performance, including the specific behaviors (or changes in behavior), strategies, measures for improvement, a timeline, and when you will meet again for a progress review.
- Obtain an explicit response from the incumbent that they understand the feedback and expected changes.

    AD: *"It's my job as the Assistant Dean for Clinical Research, and your direct supervisor, to provide you feedback on your performance. In this case, for you to be more successful with the team, I'd like to see you reduce the amount of check-in's you have with the team from multiple times a day to twice a week. I'd also like to see you come from curiosity when conducting these meetings, asking your team members how things are going and what you could do to help them, rather than, as you indicated, just telling them what to do.*

    Let's include this topic in our next monthly meeting and assess progress. I anticipate with a change in your behavior, there will be fewer complaints, and more importantly, I anticipate the members of your team will appreciate the change. I will also speak to a few of the team members over the next 3 months to see how it's going for them. How does that sound to you? Is there anything you need from me, or that I can help you with to be successful with these changes?"

The leader can make difficult conversations less so by maintaining positive regard and an optimistic tone, being clear and concise, listening consciously, providing timely feedback based on observable data, addressing behaviors that can be changed, and ensuring the incumbent has the knowledge and skills necessary to adjust and meet expectations.

Number and Format of Meetings

Typically, a first meeting can and should be more informal between just the leader and the incumbent. However, you should record notes regarding the process and content of the meeting. A second informal meeting between just the leader and incumbent might also be valuable for a "progress check" and any necessary clarification.

The goals for difficult conversations (especially pertaining to performance) should routinely include having a better understanding between the parties, improved or adjusted performance, and success for the individual(s) and organization. Logically, three general outcomes might follow an initial difficult conversation:

1. Complete resolution and maximally improved performance
2. Partial resolution with some improvement (in a given time frame)
3. Denial the problem exists or no improvement

With any of these outcomes, a follow-up meeting is always in order, but the tone and format of the meeting will be determined based on which of the outcomes occur. If complete resolution is attained the meeting can have a more informal tone, during which as leader you express your satisfaction in the outcome and thank the incumbent for learning from the situation and taking positive steps to resolve the conflict.

However, if only partial resolution or performance improvement is met, or if the incumbent refuses accountability for the issue, as the leader you should conduct a more formal meeting and engage others in the academic medical center to participate. This will likely include a representative from Human Resources, who can assist in conveying performance requirements, and the formal consequences for failing to meet previously communicated expectations. The format of this type of meeting requires considerable preparation to develop a specific communication plan and meeting strategy.

Don't Be Intimidated or Undermined

Let's face it, having difficult conversations can be intimidating. But it can be even more so if the conversation needs to occur with an employee or colleague who is older (chronologically) or more senior (in experience or years of service to the organization) to the new leader. The incumbent might try to unnerve the new leader, vocalizing their discontent, suggest an accusation is unfair, or challenge (privately, publicly, or both) the new leader's right or capacity to engage the circumstance. These are intimidation tactics.

We are not suggesting all older or more experienced members of the unit will try to intimidate you. But you should always be prepared that these behaviors could occur. If and when they do, react calmly and professionally, and adhere to the steps above. Don't let the incumbent take you down a "rabbit hole," by asking you to tell them exactly who said what, or whether you're also talking about this to someone else, or any number of diversionary tactics people can employ. Simply repeat your concerns and reiterate the unacceptable performance. Pause the conversation, if need be, and schedule a follow-up conversation for a time in the near future.

Additionally, we strongly recommend informing your supervisor you plan to have a difficult conversation *before* doing so. Additionally, provide a timely summation afterwards. Being in alignment with your supervisor helps create a unified front, should the incumbent choose to go "over your head" to complain (another intimidation tactic).

Concluding Thoughts

Effectively engaging in conflict resolution, negotiation, and mediation is critically important for all leaders. These skills and techniques can be practiced and refined through progressive experience. To continually improve, spend time in reflection after each engagement, processing outcomes, successes, and areas for development. Consider how your behaviors (words, tone, body language, etc.) may have been perceived by the other party, which behaviors you should hone, and which you should change. Pay particular attention to behaviors that evoked a significant emotional response from the other party, as well as what triggered an emotional response in you.

How Do I Get Started?

We encourage you to consider formal training courses related to these areas. Check with your Dean's Office, Human Resources, the Provost's Office, or other professional providers on your campus. People who are effective at these activities seldom do things by accident. If you have the chance to watch effective leaders utilizing these skills in action (or perhaps even participate with them), be mindful of the things they say and do, and add their techniques into your armamentarium.

Coaching questions to ask yourself:
- What about these processes seems most comfortable to me, and what parts are most uncomfortable?
- What is it that makes me uncomfortable?
- How would it make my job better if I were great at these skills?
- When I have been on the receiving end of a good negotiation, mediation, or conflict resolution, what made it go well?
- If I could get 10% better at one of these skills, what would be different for me? What do I need on work on first?
- Who do I know that is good at these skills that I can observe and learn from?

Curious to learn more?
1. Fisher R, Ury W. 2nd Ed. 1991. Getting to Yes. Penguin Books, New York, NY.
2. Hamilton, D. M. 2013. Everything is Workable. Shambhala.
3. Grenny, J., Patterson, K., McMillan, R., Switzler, A., & Gregory, E. 2021 3rd Edition. Crucial Conversations: Tools for Talking When Stakes are High. McGraw Hill.
4. Stone, D., Patton, B., Heen, S. 2010 2nd Edition. Difficult Conversations: How to Discuss What Matters Most. Penguin Books, USA.
5. Tannen D. 1990. You Just Don't Understand: Women and Men in Conversation. HarperCollins Publishers Inc. New York, NY.

References

1. Shonk K. What is conflict resolution, and how does it work? How to manage conflict at work through conflict resolution. Harvard Law School Daily Blog; 2021, December 28. Accessible at: https://www.pon.harvard.edu/daily/conflict-resolution/what-is-conflict-resolution-and-how-does-it-work/

2. Doyle A. Conflict resolution: definition, process, skills, Examples. The Balance Careers Blog; 2021, May 25. Accessible at https://www.thebalancecareers.com/conflict-resolutions-skills-2063739#citation-

3. Fisher R, Ury W. 1991. Getting to yes. Penguin Books, New York, NY. 2nd Ed.

4. Ibid, p. 42.

5. Kandell E. Workplace conflict and tone of voice. Alternative Resolutions. Available at https://www.alternativeresolutions.net/2019/02/11/workplace-conflict-and-tone-of-voice/

6. Kramer R. Stealth coaching: a roadmap to develop independent thinkers, proactive problem solvers, and exceptional leaders. 2nd ed. Eugene, OR: Luminare Press; 2020.

Crisis Leadership in the Academic Medical Center

18

There are many real and significant crises facing academic medical centers and higher education. A number stem from the COVID-19 pandemic, others from a heightened awareness of systemic racism, as well as the current political climate. Additionally, scandals, cover-ups, and other people-driven crises have taken their toll [1–3]. Healthcare and higher education have been confronted with crises including, but not limited to:

- Workforce shortages
- A growing resistance to the scientific, academic, and medical communities
- Moral trauma and burnout in the workforce
- The significant presence of mental and behavioral health challenges

For the purposes of this chapter, we have chosen to focus specifically on the types of crises the emerging leader might be confronted with in an academic medical center. "Crisis management" or "crisis leadership" remain the general terms for how organizations and leaders address critical situations, although we readily acknowledge that these can be rather insignificant in comparison to the many crises occurring throughout the world.

Crises in the academic medical center share a number of related characteristics, in that they:

- are generally unexpected and unpredictable,
- most often have a "negative" outcome,
- represent some type of "threat" to individuals, the organization, or both,
- require an immediate, deliberate response, and
- require a longer-term intervention, as the organization works to address the consequences and installs preventative strategies.

K. P. Meyer, R. Kramer, *Taking the Lead*,
https://doi.org/10.1007/978-3-031-16711-9_18

Although unexpected and intermittent, it is important that the emerging leader learns to anticipate crises. While by no means an exhaustive list, the types of crises an emerging leader in an academic medical center may face could include things such as:

- Managing research misconduct (e.g., fabrication, falsification, plagiarism)
- Mass resignation of a group of faculty or healthcare providers
- Particularly contentious student dismissal hearing
- Revelations of sexual misconduct
- Disgruntled parent registering a complaint on behalf of their adult (over 18-year-old) student
- Controversial social media posting or dispute in the news media
- Purposeful or inadvertent disclosure of protected health information
- Serious injury or unexpected death of a member of the academic medical center.[1]

A Crisis Is Coming

A crisis in the academic medical center can arise from anywhere, at any time, the result of internal or external events. This is not a "doomsday" scenario. Rather, as the leader it is vital you understand and be prepared for a crisis to occur.

As noted earlier, crisis management, or crisis leadership, is a growing yet normative and principal role of the academic medical center leader. We prefer the latter term as it speaks to the leader's role in addressing the pressing, intermediate, *and* long-term consequences of a given crisis, as well as the notion that leaders will continually confront crises.

In this regard, the question is not whether a crisis will occur, but rather if it will be appropriately addressed and learned from. If not, it risks eroding the organization, tearing away at its fabric of integrity and responsibility. We highly encourage you to be a crisis leader, staying attentive to the environment and having procedures in place to respond quickly, accurately, and effectively when a crisis occurs. This alertness also includes developing swift decision-making and follow-up skills, elevating your unit's accountability and resolve against future crises.

---

[1] Behavioral and mental health crises have become all too prevalent in academic medical centers, some regrettably resulting in suicide. Many academic medical centers have established specific crisis management teams for prevention, early identification, and treatment of mental health crises. In addition, many are implementing postvention plans and teams to provide the structure and resources for immediate and longer-term support in the aftermath of suicide. We strongly recommend new leaders familiarize themselves with the mental health crisis management teams and plans available at their academic medical center, including the crisis management phone number or contact information for a single point of contact.

Strategies and Skills for Crisis Leadership

No one wants a crisis. It's natural to want to avoid them, as crises involve people - who can get hurt, lose their jobs, have their reputations tainted, or their career plans significantly altered. We do not wish these outcomes on anybody. Yet, avoidance puts the leader and the organization in peril. We encourage you to address crises head on. As the leader, the health and welfare of your unit and the organization depend on your ability to do so. And while we certainly hope your leadership journey does not include confronting a crisis, we doubt this is realistic. Instead, recognize that the leader's journey will call for you to periodically lead through crises. It's the only way to really get better at it. As Franklin D. Roosevelt noted, "a smooth sea never made a skilled sailor."

There are many published articles and models, outlining the "phases" of crisis management and the action steps associated with each [4–7]. It is not the intent of this chapter to review these studies, nor to propose a particular preferred model. Suffice it to say, all have similar elements addressing what happens and what to do before, during, and after a crisis, often represented by the general phases of preparation, response, and follow-up.

The phases can also be divided into specific segments. For example, depending on the exact crises, the response phase may include an immediate response, as well as subsequent, early mitigating action steps. Similarly, the follow-up phase might include initial recovery, as well as long-term adaptation.

Here are a few general strategies to consider as you prepare for and lead through a crisis:

- When confronted with a crisis, be purposeful about managing your emotional response, including your own fears and uncertainty. It can be both helpful and cathartic to acknowledge your concerns (fear, self-doubt, etc.) to yourself and your close confidants, but remember you are still the leader. Everyone is looking to you for a response. So, while you may confront your own trepidation privately, do your best to exhibit calm and poise in public.[2]
- Consult with your supervisor(s), executive cabinet, or other close confidants to assist you in developing your plan and response. Be aware, the goal is to be a leader, not a "Lone Ranger."[3] A crisis is not something you should try to manage alone, nor think you need to have all the ideas and solutions.
- Develop several iterations of the initial crisis management plan. Crises tend to *unfold* rather than present all at once. At the outset, you may only be aware of the "tip of the iceberg." It is important to be facile and adaptive as you gather more

---

[2] A crisis can create a tremendous amount of uncertainty. See Chap. 6 on the negative impact this can cause.

[3] The Lone Ranger was a popular, mid-twentieth century television show, which depicted a masked, former Texas Ranger who fought outlaws. The show always ended with a shot of the Lone Ranger riding off into the sunset, an iconic image of the hero who goes it alone.

information. Be prepared to alter or even abandon your initial plan as the situation unfolds.

- Conduct an initial "threat assessment" to understand the immediate issue(s), damage (if it has occurred), and determine what mitigating and communication actions need to occur, and in what order. You may benefit from having a small group of trusted confidants assist in this endeavor. Trust those in your circle to handle parts of the information gathering and rollout. This is not the time to micromanage.
- Be as thorough as possible in gathering facts, and as contemplative in your decision-making as time permits. Remember, however, that in a crisis time is compressed, so you may not have as much of it as you'd like to make a decision. Additionally, things seldom improve in a crisis by letting time pass.[4]
- Be decisive, but not declarative. In other words, make your best decision based on the information at hand, but understand that as the crisis unfolds new information may come to light. Be cautious about making definitive or declarative statements that may need to be recanted later or that may back you into a corner.
- Time permitting, role play difficult conversations or public statements with a confidant or your executive team. You would be amazed at what you will learn and how much more confident you will feel when the real time comes.
- Recognize the tendency to "hunker down" until you have all the information and/or have formulated a comprehensive plan, but *don't do it*. Instead, be as precise as possible and communicate something as soon as possible. As more information becomes available, communicate again (and again, and again). Clear, short, and frequent communication is the key. Waiting too long to give a response may send a message that you are not in control, may not know what to do, or may be hiding something.
- During a crisis, you'll likely not have bandwidth to consider what skills you would like to work on. We said that to get better at crisis leadership, you need to lead through a crisis. Afterwards you can reflect on what went well and what could be improved upon. Thus, before you are confronted with the next crisis, be explicit with yourself about what skill(s) you are going to refine. For example, if in your last crisis you did not feel you communicated with confidence, review the associated competencies, and attempt to improve your communication approach. Pro tip: it's best to work on improving only one or two things at a time during a crisis!

The Great Multiplier

A crisis is a multiplier. Systems that have long needed improvement, ineffective policies that should have long ago been modified, or interpersonal problems that have been avoided, may all worsen in the midst of a crises. The result can be a crisis

---

[4] Understanding the limits of decision-making as described in Chap. 9 may prove helpful in this regard.

on top of a crisis, as the leader deals not only with the primary issue but also with associated weaknesses or problems that become exposed. A crisis puts stress on the organization, revealing all its cracks.

The good news is the opposite is also true. If you have good systems, policies, and relationships in place, you and your unit will be better able to withstand a crisis and effectively manage the consequences. So, take the time to address the "cracks" in your unit when times are good and calm.

Effective crisis leadership is about being proactive, not reactive. Crises are great motivators for change. Perhaps you have heard the expression, "never let a crisis go to waste." The point being, what did you learn and how will you improve going forward? Answering these questions require the leader's accountability, transparency, and tenacity. This process will likely help the unit to survive the next crisis and advance in its wake.

Toward this end, we also suggest:

- After a crisis has ended, conduct a post-mortem, "plus/delta" review to determine what you did well (plus) and what you could improve upon (delta). Not long after the event is resolved, make the necessary changes. Don't wait. Get the professional development you and others need and collectively discuss the learnings that can applied to the next crisis.
- Training and coaching can be exceptionally helpful. Be purposeful about any new knowledge or competencies you develop so you can be sure to put them in to practice when the next event occurs.
- Consider whether there was an underlying cause to the crises that could have been identified sooner, or that necessitates a policy, procedural, or personnel change, and make the appropriate adaptations.

It's important to be deliberate about starting and completing these actions. It is not unusual for the immediate sense of urgency to give way to the status quo. The result being the leader and unit remain unprepared, having missed a major improvement opportunity for handling the next crisis.

However, leaders that do examine lessons learned seize the opportunity to hit the organization's reset button. They recognize that present turbulence can force change to key rules of the game, reshaping parts of the organization, and redefining the work the unit does. Leaders who do this are said to practice *adaptive leadership* [8, 9], a critical skill using a growth mindset to effectively adjust to and manage situations effectively. In this case, the leader adjusts well to a crisis to continually improve the unit or organization.

How Do I Get Started?

Managing a crisis is not for the faint of heart and becoming adept at crisis leadership takes perseverance and a willingness to continually learn and grow. But once you begin to have your arms around it, you will find that it is another important part of the leader's job. Understand too, that along with learning how to effectively deal with crises, you will likely learn a multitude of other skills, such as priority management, establishing healthy boundaries, self-care, and vulnerability/asking for help. This is all good and important growth. Leadership is a moving Venn diagram of hundreds of skills. And a crisis brings many needed leadership skills into play at once.

Coaching questions to ask yourself:
- What concerns me most about my ability to effectively lead through a crisis?
- When I am stressed, what happens to my abilities to lead? Is there anything I need to be aware of or self-regulate?
- How can I get better at this competency?
- What other significant challenges have I overcome in my career? How did I go about getting better with managing those?
- Who have I witnessed leading well through a crisis? What did they do and say that gave me this impression?

Curious to learn more?
1. Cowen, S. S. (2018, August 13). Shared Governance Does Not Mean Shared Decision Making. The Chronicle of Higher Education. https://www.chronicle.com/article/shared-governance-does-not-mean-shared-decision-making/
2. Heifetz, R. (2019). Leadership in a (Permanent) Crisis. Harvard Business Review; Harvard Business Publishing. https://hbr.org/2009/07/leadership-in-a-permanent-crisis
3. Jacques, T. (2014). Issue and crisis management: exploring issues, crises, risk and reputation. Oxford Press.
4. Kramer, R. (2020, May 22). Looking on the Bright Side of Life. Inside Higher Ed; Inside Higher Ed. https://www.insidehighered.com/advice/2020/05/22/some-suggested-tactics-leading-during-trying-time-opinion
5. Marker, A. (2020, July 20). Proactive vs Reactive Crisis Management Model. Smartsheet. https://www.smartsheet.com/content/crisis-management-model-theories
6. Spierling, K., & Palmer, J. (2020, November 6). The Time for Teamwork Is Now. Inside Higher Ed; Inside Higher Ed. https://www.insidehighered.com/advice/2020/11/06/professor-and-administrator-provide-advice-effectively-working-teams-opinion
7. Zdziarski, E. L. (Ed.). (2020). *Campus Crisis Management*. Routledge.

Watch a movie filled with crisis leadership examples:
8. Howard, R. (Director). (1995). *Apollo 13* [Film]. Imagine Entertainment.

References

1. Lacey E, Wolcott R. Timeline: Michigan state and its handling of sexual assault cases. Lansing State J. 2018, March 27; Available at https://www.lansingstatejournal.com/story/news/local/2018/03/27/michigan-state-university-timeline/336540002/
2. Chappell B. NPR KIOS; 2012, July 21. Available at https://www.npr.org/2011/11/08/142111804/penn-state-abuse-scandal-a-guide-and-timeline
3. Full Coverage: The college admissions scheme. Los Angeles Times. Available at https://www.latimes.com/california/story/la-me-college-admissions-storygallery
4. Chadha P. The four phases of crisis management. AGB Blog Post; 2020, October 6. Available at https://agb.org/blog-post/the-four-phases-of-crisis-management/
5. Institute for Public Relations. Crisis management and communications. 2007, October 30. Available at https://instituteforpr.org/crisis-management-and-communications/#:~:text=Crisis%20 management%20can%20be%20divided,actually%20respond%20to%20a%20crisis.
6. Go MH. Identify the stages of a crisis. Business Continuity Management Institute (BCM) Blog. 2021, June 28.; Available at https://blog.bcm-institute.org/crisis-management/identify-the-stages-of-a-crisis
7. Pedersen CL, Ritter T, Di Benedetto CA. Managing through a crisis: managerial implications for business-to-business firms. Ind Mark Manag. 2020;88:314–22. https://doi.org/10.1016/j.indmarman.2020.05.034.
8. Heifetz R. Leadership in a (Permanent) crisis. Harvard Business Review; Harvard Business Publishing; 2019. Available at https://hbr.org/2009/07/leadership-in-a-permanent-crisis
9. Ramalingam B, et al. 5 Principles to guide adaptive leadership. Harvard Business Rev. 2020, September 11; https://hbr.org/2020/09/5-principles-to-guide-adaptive-leadership

Betrayal: Such Is the Life of a Leader

19

A trusted colleague breaks the confidence of a co-worker. Someone takes credit for another's idea. A supervisor promises an employee a new role or promotion only to give it to someone else. A faction in a unit attempts to discredit the success of their colleague. Regrettably, these are common examples of workplace betrayal.

What we write about in this chapter is a specific type of betrayal, however. Namely the leader being betrayed by a trusted colleague. Betrayal is not an inevitability that all leaders will experience. However, we believe it is important that leaders have an explicit understanding that it can and does happen. Therefore, it is vital that the new leader understands betrayal, can recognize its early warning signs, and develops strategies for effectively addressing a betrayal.

Leadership Betrayal

At its core, betrayal is about broken trust, when someone who is a principal and close colleague (even friend), turns on you. When it occurs, it can be a very personal, even painful event. And if not dealt with properly, it can also derail your leadership career.

There may be any number of reasons a trusted colleague chooses to betray a leader. Ambition, impatience, or insecurity might be at play. If you take on a leadership role within your academic medical center, a former peer might view your success as undeserved, or relatedly that they (not you) are the reason for your success. Consequently, they may feel undervalued and underappreciated. It's also not unusual in hierarchical organizations such as academic medical centers for the leader to receive accolades for the unit's success. In such a case, the betrayer may perceive the leader's recognition as unjustified. Ultimately, the betrayer comes to overvalue themselves and undervalue the leader's role.

Once feeling embittered, the betrayer may begin to misrepresent information provided by the leader. They may filter or alter what they communicate to others, constructing an alternate reality, or driving their own personal agenda. The betrayer

© The Author(s), under exclusive license to Springer Nature Switzerland AG 2022
K. P. Meyer, R. Kramer, *Taking the Lead*,
https://doi.org/10.1007/978-3-031-16711-9_19

may create a narrative for themselves, believing that they alone possess the knowledge or capability to realize the unit's vision. They may become progressively outspoken and emboldened, or increasingly secretive. They may either gain followers who they influence to feel similarly, or become increasingly isolated. It can be hard for the new leader to decipher what is happening in these moments. We encourage the leader to pay close attention when a colleague is suddenly gaining or losing informal followership.

In addition, early signs of pending betrayal may be the colleague who becomes progressively impatient and disenchanted with the leader, their vision, or their promises. The duplicity often comes to full fruition when the betrayer chooses to deploy some form of retribution, usually disparaging the leader's reputation or spreading disinformation about the unit.

The "Storyline" of Betrayal

What makes the action described above even more disheartening is that at one time the betrayer was supportive of the leader's choices and vision. Often the betrayer comes to believe that the leader has lost sight of their original vision or is not progressing fast enough, thus blaming the leader for the betrayal (implying it was necessary for the benefit of the unit). However, the betrayal is typically the result of a change in the *betrayer* (though they would seldom recognize or admit this).

The "story" of betrayal generally includes several common elements. First, the relationship between the leader and the colleague begins in a positive manner, often beginning as a professional relationship, and even becoming a personal friendship. In the case of the academic medical center, it is common for the leader to have been personally involved in the recruitment of the colleague, and perhaps also served as a mentor or collaborator. The roles are also sometimes reversed, and the colleague had originally helped to recruit the new leader.

Based on the development of this strong relationship, it would not be unusual for the colleague to at some point serve alongside the leader, exerting a relatively high degree of influence in the unit, either as a recognized "informal" leader, or in a formal leadership role. The leader likely provided considerable development opportunities for the colleague, advocated on their behalf, and may have even defended them if a difficult situation arose.

At some point during the relationship, however, things begin to take a detour, for any number of ostensible reasons. The leader begins to notice the colleague drifting away. Based on the quality and depth of the relationship, the leader may feel comfortable to query the colleague regarding these perceptions. Oftentimes the colleague denies that anything is wrong or attributes their behavior to some other vague source.

At some point one of two outcomes are likely to occur: either (1) disruptive or disengaging behaviors begin to escalate, or (2) the colleague becomes withdrawn and secretive. They may express a desire to investigate other employment opportunities (within or outside of the institution). They may become more demanding, indicating their value to the unit and organization, and requesting a salary increase or other resources or recognition. Interestingly, it is not unusual for the leader to meet these requests, or at least attempt to do so in some manner. The leader may not yet fully comprehend the beginning of the betrayal, or they may have an incorrect assumption (or hope) that meeting the requests will reengage the colleague.

This "retention strategy" might salvage the relationship. But if the betrayer is truly disgruntled, it will likely only result in a few months of the colleague being placated. If bent on betrayal, at some point the colleague will likely make an abrupt, declarative decision. They may indicate the leader's support was insufficient, or they may even deny the additional support was given at all. They may publicly indicate displeasure with the leader or the unit. Often, they pull the desperate move of announcing their intent to leave the organization, hoping that will shift things greatly in their favor.

Were the story to stop here, we would not consider it to be one of betrayal. It would be the unfortunate tale of a disgruntled employee who ultimately decided to leave the unit. In the "betrayal" story line, however, there is one more significant element. After the individual plays their final card (announces they will be resigning), they decide to "go public."

This usually takes the form of expressing their discontent to everyone they know, disparaging and spreading disinformation about the leader, and often blaming the leader for their now "necessary" departure. They may even take their concerns to senior executives in the organization or write a diatribe in their employment exit survey. These behaviors may or may not be brought to the leader's attention in time to mitigate the impact. But at some point, the leader will learn the betrayer tried to "burn the place down" on the way out the door, attempting to ruin the reputation of the leader and potentially the unit. *This is the substance of a betrayal story.*

Results of Betrayal

It is important to note that most leaders may never experience this depth of disloyalty, or if they do, only rarely. We don't want to be too melodramatic or Shakespearian here. But if it does happen, it can have a significant impact on the leader as well as the unit.

For the leader, there is the emotional turmoil associated with a close colleague and friend turning against them. The leader may experience any number of reactions in response to a betrayal. Bewilderment, anger at the betrayer, and perhaps consideration of retribution are common reactions. The leader may also assume unnecessary responsibility for the events. They may be upset with themselves for missing something in the relationship, having been too trusting, not being able to effectively "read people," or thinking they may have caused the betrayer's actions.

These thoughts and emotions can shake the leader's confidence and cause them to question their abilities. Engaging in conversation with supervisors, friends, loved ones, or even a therapist can be of great assistance. Coaching may also be valuable during this time, assisting the leader in systematic reflection, proper reframing of the event(s), and the creation of a plan to move forward.

Beyond dealing with their personal emotions, the leader may also need to assess any reputational damage the betrayer caused with members of the unit or the organization. Conversations with others may be in order, but be clear, the goal of these exchanges is not for the leader to defend themselves or attempt to repudiate the claims of the betrayer. The leader must remain professional and should avoid the temptation to blame or disparage the betrayer. If others raise concerns about what the betrayer may have told them, the leader can use the opportunity to correct the disinformation, and if appropriate, express any insights into what could have been done more effectively. More importantly, the leader can provide assurances they are doing well and are as committed as ever to their role and to the success of the unit. In the end, there is a limit to how wide a net the leader should cast in determining reputational damage, as it can be consuming to the point of it being unhealthy.

As we noted, betrayal is oftentimes a "public event," so members of the unit have likely seen the event unfold and may be affected by the disruption and uncertainty. In this circumstance, the leader needs to focus less on the details of the betrayal, and more on addressing any concerns the members have, as well as assuring them the unit remains highly functional. The leader needs to re-emphasize their commitment to leading the unit and its members to success. Because the "news cycle" is relatively short in the academic medical center, in most instances, any reputational concerns will dissipate fairly quickly if the leader remains positive and focused on the unit's success.

How to Respond to Betrayal

One purpose in writing this chapter was to alert you to the fact that betrayal can occur. But it is not inevitable. If you notice early warning signs, or an abrupt shift in the quality of your relationship with a previously trusted colleague, speak with them. The tone of this conversation should be curious, not accusatory. Inquire about their general well-being and if they have any concerns. You can cite the behaviors you have noted and inquire about their purpose or intent, noting what you consider to be unintended outcomes that perhaps they had not realized. For instance, you may note their recent increase in open dissent during unit meetings, pointing out it is both different than their "usual" behavior, and that it has had the effect of limiting input from other members of the unit.

You might also note the general change in the person's attitude or engagement toward you. Ask if they have noticed the same, and whether you did or said anything that may have contributed to this change. Be alert to your own emotional reaction, as you may get constructive but difficult feedback. Avoid the temptation to become defensive, and indicate you appreciate the feedback and will take it under advisement. Finish the conversation with a plan to meet again to continue the discussion.

A word of caution here. A conversation like this can go one of two ways. It can open up a much-needed dialogue, where the leader and colleague engage constructively, restoring the relationship or making it even more effective. Or it can "cement" the colleague's contrarian views and plans. Bear in mind, if the colleague's ultimate strategy is leaving the institution, this may actually be a good outcome in the end. On the other hand, if the colleague views the conversation as the leader "forcing" them to resign, they may subsequently consider forms of retribution.

If the problems exist largely in the mind of the colleague, and the circumstances have reached the point of open dissent, generally there is little opportunity to bring the wayward individual back into the fold. It is likely best at this point for the betrayer to move on. Unfortunately, any number of circumstances, not the least of which might be inertia, may keep the betrayer from resigning. Consequently, it may be in the best interest of the leader and the organization to actively pursue resignation or termination. Not doing so will likely allow the betrayer to become progressively more destructive to the unit, if not the entire organization.

If resignation or termination is an option, we recommend you work with your human resources department to either impose an administrative leave between the decision point of resignation and the actual date of resignation, or if possible, make the resignation effective immediately (even if there is a payout involved). This strategy will limit the betrayer's access to people and information, helping diminish or mitigate attempts at reprisal.

Situations Not to Be Confused as Betrayal

As a new leader, you will encounter a number of unique situations that may at first appear to include betrayal. Though these situations may contain "elements" of betrayal, we want to be clear they are *not* betrayal. Recognizing and responding appropriately is critical to each of the examples below.

For starters you will meet people in the academic medical center who do not like you. The reasons seldom matter in the long run. People who don't like you may be less than enthusiastic about working with you. They may even oppose parts of your work, but they are *not* betraying you. They just don't like you. Sometimes, if you're willing to put in the effort, you can mend these relationships and win these individuals over. Regardless, you'll need to develop strategies to work effectively with them.

Similarly, betrayal should not be confused with periodic disagreements you will likely have with others. Not everyone will agree with every decision you make, and thus, disagreements and conflict are part of the fabric of leadership. If the parties involved exhibit good will, disagreements are generally resolvable. And, at times, you will need to move forward with a decision even in the face of disagreement.

Another related circumstance is an employee who comes to you to indicate dissatisfaction with their work (duties, work volume, salary, etc.). This is a legitimate conversation to have. If you ask the employee how their situation might improve, they may request your help with solving a problem, providing a salary increase, redistributing their work duties, etc. These may or may not be requests that you can accommodate.

The employee may also indicate they have an outside job offer that they are strongly considering unless one of the aforementioned actions is taken. In deciding whether to pursue a course of action to retain the employee, the leader should consider such things as the employee's productivity as a member of the team, the amount of disruption their departure would have on others, how difficult it would be to replace the employee, and the impact a salary increase, or work redistribution would have on the unit.

If you deem their concerns to be credible and you desire to retain the employee, we suggest you make every effort to do so, *once*. However, we recommend you not let this strategy become a recurring event. If you are approached by the same employee a second time with similar concerns or demands, and again with the "threat" of leaving the organization, it may be time for you to support them taking the new role and wish them well in their new pursuits. This situation is not betrayal, but rather an employee wanting a particular course of action or special treatment that you may not be able to, or choose not to, accommodate.

Lastly, you may have a high performing employee that you also have a positive relationship with who chooses to leave for another opportunity. This happens all the time in academic medical centers. Their departure may simply reflect a positive outcome, that you are supporting the success of your team and that they are ready for their next career challenges. It could also be a sign, however, that the unit or organization needs to provide more growth opportunities and better retention strategies. Or it could be that the departing employee wanted to move closer to family. In any case, this is not betrayal, it's simply life.

Learning from Betrayal

Hopefully, you will not encounter betrayal in your leadership journey. Yet by recognizing that it can happen, and being aware of the early warning signs, perhaps you will be able to either restore the relationship or diminish negative outcomes before they occur. Remember too, as time passes, usually any results of a betrayal will fade, as does the pain you experienced.

It's wise to evaluate a betrayal event for what can be learned from it, but we recommend this not occur too soon after the event. The best time to conduct a "postmortem" is several weeks (or longer) after it occurred. This will allow the leader time to let any emotions subside (theirs or others') and regain their own confidence. Allowing some distance from the event will also help the leader realistically evaluate the value of the former relationship, what they learned from it, and whether there was anything they might have done differently.

Work to identify any "early warning signs" from the event should they occur again. Consider the conditions under which the betrayal occurred. These may have only impacted the betrayer the last time, but there may have been broader organizational or unit-based circumstances that contributed and need to be addressed going forward.

If you experience a betrayal as a leader, understand that you may be a little "leery" trusting others for a while. That's reasonable, maybe even to be expected. Despite these feelings, we encourage you to go through this evaluation process, and recommend you do so with the guidance of a supervisor, mentor, or coach. The goal of this assessment is no different than any other leadership development process. Build awareness (of the potential signs of betrayal), work on any areas identified for your improvement, and create a plan for proactively moving forward. Take ownership and make necessary improvements (to the conditions and/or your leadership skills), but don't beat yourself up. Remember, you don't cause people to betray you, they choose to do so. The closure afforded by an assessment process will help you not become jaded, and to continue to trust others.

While perhaps easier said than done, we encourage you to "forgive and forget." The world of academic medical centers is relatively small, so it's likely you'll run into your betrayer at a future point in time, perhaps at a professional meeting, on a national committee, or even working again at the same institution. At the very least, determine an effective strategy to limit your engagement with your former betrayer, exhibit grace for what happened in the past, and move on. In the end, honor your integrity and keep your head held high.

How Do I Get Started?

The shock of a workplace betrayal can take its toll. We encourage you to have resources and strategies for managing stress, and perhaps trauma. A favorite book to consider is Pema Chodron's, "When Things Fall Apart" (see below). This short but powerful read provides effective reflections and tools on dealing with life's most difficult moments. It is a book co-author, Rob, will often recommend to his coaching clients.

Coaching questions to ask yourself:
- What is the story I am currently telling myself about this betrayal?
- What is a new way I could tell this story that helps me learn and grow as a leader?
- How have I managed setbacks in the past (professionally or personally), and what can I learn from those experiences?
- What aspects of this betrayal sting the most, and why?
- What can I hold myself accountable for in this situation, and what do I need to let go of or let the betrayer own?
- What do I need to move past this event in a healthy way?

Curious to learn more?
1. Betrayed in the Workplace? 7 Steps for Healing. Center for Creative Leadership. Available at https://www.ccl.org/articles/leading-effectively-articles/betrayed-workplace-7-steps-healing/
2. Carucci, R. What to Do When Your Boss Betrays You. July 23, 2019. Harvard Business Review. Available at https://hbr.org/2019/07/what-to-do-when-your-boss-betrays-you
3. Chodron, P. (2016). When Things Fall Apart: Heart Advice for Difficult Times. Shambhala.
4. Martell G. Betrayed at Work? Here's How to Move Forward in Your Career. Elevatework.com. Available at https://www.ellevatenetwork.com/articles/10848-betrayed-at-work-here-s-how-to-move-forward-in-your-career
5. Praslova, L. N. (2022, January 14). Feeling distressed at work? It might be more than burnout. Fast Company; Fast Company. https://www.fastcompany.com/90712671/feeling-distressed-at-work-it-might-be-more-than-burnout
6. Redden, E. (2021, November 12). Researching 'Institutional Courage.' Inside Higher Ed; Inside Higher Ed. https://www.insidehighered.com/news/2021/11/12/center-funds-research-institutional-courage
7. Twibell, R., & Townsend, T. (2011, November 11). Trust in the workplace: Build it, break it, mend it. American Nurse; American Nurse. https://www.myamericannurse.com/trust-in-the-workplace-build-it-break-it-mend-it/

Part V

Epilogue

You Can't Lead if You Don't Take Care of Yourself

20

Leadership is more than a full-time job, it's a lifestyle. You never really get away from your role as leader. Consequently, it's important for leaders to have other interests. Such things will keep you physically and emotionally healthy and better able to handle the daily grind of leadership work. You may also be amazed what you learn from your other interests that you can bring to your leadership role.

There's More to Life than Leading

Author, Kyle's, hobby is biking. When he tells people "I'm a biker," they get this peculiar look on their face… he can see the bubble over their head and hear them saying to themselves, "You?! A skinny, old guy like you, on a Harley?" Based on that quizzical look, he often follows with the correction, "No, I mean I'm a bicyclist." At which point he envisions their unspoken response to be, "Ohhh… a skinny, old guy wearing spandex padded shorts, and a goofy helmet, well that makes perfect sense." Author, Rob's, experience is not so dissimilar to Kyle's, as a longtime bicyclist as well, though perhaps a little less "old!"

Bicycling as a Metaphor for Leadership

We want to share some lessons learned about being a leader—from bicycling—to illustrate the value of applying other interests to your own leadership. Let's start with the aforementioned padded shorts. No offense if you're also a bicyclist, but in our opinion, there are few, if any, sports where the "uniform" required for participation is more dreadful than bicycling. On the list of the "top 100 coolest uniforms" (if such a list exists), bicycling gear would be #101, just below the wrestling singlet (apologies to any former wrestlers).

K. P. Meyer, R. Kramer, *Taking the Lead*,
https://doi.org/10.1007/978-3-031-16711-9_20

Bicycle "bibs" are essentially a wrestling singlet equipped with a large foam diaper sewn in to protect one's nether regions on long rides in the saddle. If you're going to be a serious bicyclist you greatly appreciate the gear. What has wearing this uniform taught us about leadership? Take your *role or function* very seriously, but don't take *yourself* too seriously.

Secondly, a bicycle is a great metaphor for the organization a leader leads. A bicyclist works *with* their bicycle to get somewhere. The bicyclist, like the leader, has three basic jobs: (1) have the destination in mind (vision), (2) steer the bicycle (provide direction), and (3) pedal (provide energy to reach the destination).

Additionally, anyone who has bicycled for more than a few miles will tell you not to hold onto the handlebars too tightly (i.e., micromanaging or over managing). If you do, you're at risk of tiring out quickly, your hands getting numb and losing your fine touch, and your arms and body being too rigid, influencing the tendency to overcorrect if you encounter unforeseen obstacles. Hopefully the application of these metaphors to leadership is obvious.

Wind, Wind, and More Wind

Here' the thing about riding a bike outdoors – there's no shortage of wind. We will delve into three types of wind, but before we do, let's establish a general "attitude" about the wind. You cannot let yourself get emotionally affected by the wind. If you do, on the days it's with you (wind at your back), you'll feel great, other days, when it's against you (in your face or blowing sideways), you'll be frustrated and/or angry. These attitudes will do nothing to change the presence of the wind, or the fact that you still have to ride in it.

To stick with biking, you'd better really like it. And the same is true of leadership. You must be aware that you will regularly encounter continual, often gusty, winds. Our advice is to simply acknowledge that there will always be wind. Don't get too high if the wind is with you, or too low if it's against you, because you can't control it, you never know when it's going to change direction, and in the end the "good" wind days and the "bad" wind days all even out.

Speaking of wind, generally, there are three kinds, (1) tailwind, a wind that blows in the direction you're moving, (2) headwind, a wind that blows against the direction you're moving, and (3) crosswind, a wind that blows perpendicular to your path. Throughout your leadership journey you'll experience each of these winds routinely. Let's examine the impact of each on our leadership ride.

A good tailwind makes riding *so easy* that the work of pedaling can seem almost effortless, as you let the wind blow you along. In professional cycling they have a term for this, "having no chain," because the riding fells so effortless it's as if you don't experience resistance, even when pedaling. But here's the paradox, when the wind is with you—when your leadership journey is going great—your supervisor is pleased with your performance, you and your colleagues are all on the same page, you feel like you're making a profound impact, everything you touch seems to succeed – *do not* just let the wind take you. Rather, *pedal like crazy.*

Remember, the wind won't always be with you, so take advantage of these times in your leadership journey when a good tailwind acts as a multiplier. Work your hardest when everything is going your way. Shift to a bigger gear and pedal as fast as you can, covering as much ground as possible to move your leadership opportunities and accomplishments forward at great speed.

On the flip side, a strong headwind is just plain horrible to ride in. Some riders advise pedaling harder into a headwind to try to maintain speed. That might be sound advice in a sprint, but remember, your ride is going to be very long. Endurance is the key. If you pedal harder into a headwind to try to overcome its effects, all you'll do is wear yourself out, and fast.

It is in these moments you need to remind yourself that the wind's direction will eventually change. If the wind is blowing directly in your face—your leadership journey seems at a standstill—perhaps you aren't seeing "eye-to-eye" with your supervisor(s) or colleagues, or you can't seem to move a project forward. You're trying your hardest, but it seems like everything you touch fails. Or frankly you're just having a stretch of time where your energy is low.

The temptation might be to get off the bike and wait for the wind to die down. Don't do that, you don't know how long it will be before the wind changes, and once you stop riding, it's hard to get started again. You might also be tempted to turn around, so the wind is at your back. We don't recommend doing that either. It is hard work to "stay the course," but even slow progression forward is better than moving back quicker over ground you've already covered.

The best advice during these times is to *stay steady*. In bicycle terms, you want to try to maintain a steady pedaling cadence (the number of revolutions of the pedals per minute). To do that though, you will need to shift the gears to make your pedaling easier and preserve energy. And that's OK. There is no shame in "just hanging in there" for a period of time until the wind changes direction. Use this steady peddling time to think, plan, and prepare, so that when the wind does change, you're ready to go. One last piece of advice about riding into a headwind: we've found it best to keep your mouth shut during these times (literally) unless you want a mouth full of bugs.[1]

Crosswinds are interesting for a couple of reasons. For one, they are annoying. We like to know when we are sailing along or when we have direct resistance, but a crosswind is sometimes hard to read because it is neither, it blows perpendicular to your path. A strong crosswind makes it hard to maintain your balance for any length of time.

Here's the interesting thing about managing a strong crosswind, you need to lean into it. Think for example that the wind is blowing from your left to right, in other words, it is pushing your bike to the right. If you don't lean to the left, you could get blown over to the right. You need to stay alert, however, because if the crosswind

---

[1] Rob once suffered the ails of this mistake and had a bee fly into his mouth. Fortunately, neither the bee nor the human was hurt as a result. Though both had a good story to tell when they got home.

changes and begins to come from the other direction, you will need to adjust and lean the other direction. Otherwise, you risk being off balancing and crashing.

Think of a crosswind as a metaphor for change. If a chapter of your leadership journey feels "out of balance," things seem confusing, or you feel like you are being pummeled from both sides, look for opportunities to make a turn—either adjust to a current crosswind to make it a headwind (at least you now know what you're dealing with), or take advantage of it, course correct, and make it a new tailwind (find opportunities amidst the chaos).

A few other pieces of advice to guide your ride:

1. Don't stop pedaling; you'll soon fall over.
2. Keep your head up to see where you're going (or perhaps more accurately, to see what's coming at you).
3. Bring hydration and snacks; fueling is essential for a long journey.
4. Be alert; never expect others (i.e., people in cars) to watch out for you.
5. Occasionally you'll need to stand up out of your seat and pedal (i.e., try something different). If you don't, your rear end is going to get mighty sore.
6. Always wear a helmet; you're probably gonna' take a few knocks to the head.

What's Your Destination?

A final piece of advice. There's an often-quoted adage about leadership, "the journey is more important than the destination." We agree that the *journey* of leadership can be amazing, enlightening, and even life changing. However, we think this quote misses a couple of key elements about leadership.

First, you need to understand the ride (your leadership journey) won't always be pretty, the road won't always be smooth, and sometimes you may be the only one on it. Second, your destination *is* important - for the members of your unit, your organization, and ultimately for you. In our view, if you don't know where you're going, what will motivate you to get up and ride every day? And more importantly, why would anyone else want to follow you? Sure, occasionally you'll have to take an alternate route, but you still need to have a plan for where you want to go. If you don't, you'll likely get lost, or worse yet, you may end up just riding in circles.

Have a Good Ride!

Our purpose in writing this epilogue was to encourage you to have avocations (i.e., interests or hobbies), outside of your leadership vocation (occupation). We believe that regardless of what your hobbies or interests are, you can draw inspiration and wisdom from them to inform and inspire your leadership calling. In fact, some of your best leadership insights might come from the least expected places. Because of our shared interest in bicycling, we had fun writing this chapter. Whether or not you're a bicyclist, we trust you recognize the sound leadership parallels between bicycling and leadership, despite some of our tongue-in-cheek observations.

On a serious note, we also want to caution you that the responsibilities of leadership can quickly and easily become all consuming. Routine self-care, time with friends and family, volunteer engagement, vacation, or any number of avocations (like bicycling) can often be the first "victims" of a singular devotion to leadership. We offer that being purposeful and deliberate about taking care of yourself is as much a responsibility of leadership as any other activity. Doing so will help you establish and maintain your effectiveness as a leader, and it will substantially increase your personal fulfillment.

The academic medical center is a tremendous asset to the U.S. healthcare system. Sustaining and expanding the potential of this entity in the decades ahead will require the next generation of great leaders. If you have read this book, we believe you are one of those leaders, and we want you to fully realize your potential and contributions. Don't let the demands and trappings of leadership overwhelm you. To the contrary, for the benefit of yourself, those you love, those you lead, the organization in which you contribute, and the community you impact, take care of yourself.

We are imagining great things!

Index

© The Editor(s) (if applicable) and The Author(s), under exclusive license to Springer
Nature Switzerland AG 2022
K. P. Meyer, R. Kramer, *Taking the Lead*, https://doi.org/10.1007/978-3-031-16711-9